FORTY FAVOURS THE BRAVE

ABOUT THE AUTHORS

Blasting onto the Australian media scene in 2017, Lise Carlaw and Sarah Wills are a duo with a difference. Their extraordinary friendship and chemistry landed the pair local and national radio shows with the largest broadcast network in the country. Walking the line between smart and irreverent, they've interviewed household names, from formidable politicians to global celebrities, in front of audiences of thousands.

In 2020, the year Lise and Sarah turned forty, they launched the podcast equivalent of a little black book for the middle years, *FORTY*. Following much success, *FORTY* celebrates the life lessons and stories of popular and everyday women in their fifth decade.

FORTY

FAVOURS THE BRAVE

Lise Carlaw & Sarah Wills

echo

echo

Echo Publishing
An imprint of Bonnier Books UK
4th Floor, Victoria House, Bloomsbury Square
London WC1B 4DA
www.echopublishing.com.au
www.bonnierbooks.co.uk

Echo Publishing acknowledges the traditional custodians of country throughout Australia. We recognise their continuing connection to land, sea and waters. We pay our respects to elders past and present.

First published 2022
Reprinted 2022

Printed and bound in Australia by Griffin Press

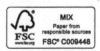

The paper this book is printed on is certified against the Forest Stewardship Council® Standards. Griffin Press holds FSC® chain of custody certification SGS-COC-005088. FSC® promotes environmentally responsible, socially beneficial and economically viable management of the world's forests.

Cover design by Evi O. Studio | Wilson Leung
Page design and typesetting by Shaun Jury

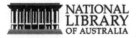

A catalogue entry for this book is available from the National Library of Australia

ISBN: 9781760686970 (paperback)
ISBN: 9781760687281 (ebook)

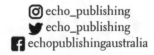
echo_publishing
echo_publishing
echopublishingaustralia

Contents

Introduction

The most curious of things happens around forty. Like a meerkat on sentry duty, you pop out of a tunnel and begin swivelling around on high alert, looking behind, around and ahead, trying to grasp the lay of the land.

It dawns how quickly the last few decades have whizzed by without you noticing; how is it possible to stand on the precipice of middle age when it feels like twenty-six was just yesterday? And if the first forty years were a retrospective blur of time marked with the ego and decisions of youth, the question is: will the remaining half of life be more of the same?

> *So much of our life we slide into – we slide into jobs, we slide into relationships, we slide into our friendships and having children. Forties is about deciding, 'I want to decide not to slide'.*
> — Angela Mollard

This is the point at which we found ourselves.

But first, let's step back in time ...

While pregnant with our respective second children (who were born two days apart in 2013), we began following each other online. For any future generations perusing our story, that may read as distinctly

1

stalker-ish, but the truth is we'd both amassed large audiences through our individual writing and musings on life, connecting with women across the world. On a resumé, we would describe this as being freelance authors, but the truth is ... we had blogs.

Sure. Look, regardless – it was a way to stay creative and hold a little pocket of space and time for ourselves while on maternity leave, muddling through life with tiny children in tow.

At thirty-three, when the babies were four months old, we finally met in the flesh; the dress code for our 'date' was pyjamas and slippers in Sarah's lounge room. Lise rocked up with a wheel of warm brie from the convenience store and it became a marathon five hours of non-stop talking and discovery. The similarities were uncanny and went far beyond being born in 1980 and living a suburb away. There were old mutual friends – one of whom invited both of us to her wedding in 2006 but Lise was living overseas, and Sarah ended up at the same table as Lise's future husband. In 2008, we married men with first names starting with D (although Sarah has called her husband 'Wills', their family name, since they met). Our mothers were born in December, our mothers-in-law were both named Ann. We had the same fertility issue (a luteal phase deficiency, which resulted in miscarriages) and were under the care of the same doctor at the same time. And on it went – from near misses during university years and model castings in the small pool that was our city.

From the very beginning, ours was the most wonderful kind of no-frills connection, and we often say we 'fell in friendship love' that night. In fact, it changed the course of our entire lives. We were catapulted into each other's every day, and so began a frantic catch-up of the younger years we missed knowing each other, which was unexpected given we both had – and continue to have – close heritage friendships spanning decades.

It's tricky to explain why there was such a burning need to know each other, and with such urgency. Each immediately understood the other – and there was a clear recognition of being creatively unfulfilled as individuals whose talents and skills had slowly faded into the background as we flailed about in the common reality of asking, 'Is this it?' in our thirties. We figuratively clung to each other like overboard sailors would a pillar buoy, before deciding to rescue ourselves.

It came one day when Lise blurted out a daydream she'd had. Nobody likes a dream story, but this one was different. Her mind's eye had wandered off to a random place where the two of us were standing on stage holding microphones. To cut a long story short, despite us having no public profile and still wearing nursing bras, Sarah thought the idea sounded solid and not at all delusional.

That was all Lise needed to hunt out an opportunity. After seeing tickets to an exclusive event screening for *The Bachelor Australia* finale, she cold called the venue manager and asked if they would perhaps enjoy the free services of an emcee duo who'd never worked onstage together before, had no prior clients under their belt, but happened to be mad fans of the series. As it turns out, Lise's call (from Sarah's back deck, with her nervously pacing around) had interrupted their planning meeting about the event, which included finding hosts. They said yes. You couldn't make this stuff up.

While serendipity was on our side, so was strategy. The simple fact is, we recognised a gap in the market for representation around female friendship. Remember, this was 2015, and while outgoing and fun male co-hosts were a dime a dozen, the same space was not held for women to be smart, natural and witty, with free-flowing banter. As a general rule, we'd noticed the women who were emceeing events were always incredibly polished and slick with popular appeal – think newsreaders and journos – who did magnificent jobs of delivering the set script but weren't afforded the same freedom to showcase their personalities the way their male counterparts were.

In hindsight, there was a bravery in two women backing themselves and unapologetically fronting up to offer a different alternative. And it worked – subsequent word-of-mouth from the 200-plus audience at *The Bachelor Australia* event resulted in a slow-but-steady stream of growth from unpaid gigs to paid client work. The first joint fee we received was $300 to host an Australian designer's VIP fashion night, and our excitement was off the charts. We had commercialised our friendship and, within a year, clients were paying up to ten times more for us to front up, on stage, with microphones. Lise's daydream had become our reality: the Those Two Girls brand and company was born.

....

Sidebar: We realise the 'Girls' element may be problematic to some as we grow older, but we chose it at the time knowing descriptions were landing at 'you know, those two girls hosted it – what are their names, Lisa or Liz-someone and Sarah?' Thanks to Lise's French heritage, it's been a constant struggle for the Aussie masses to understand her name rhymes with cheese, trees, please and fleas. Hence, we are Those Two Girls forevermore thanks to its humorous origin at a moment in time – it's not politically correct, but Lise's name is a cross we bear. It also cost us $10,000 to trademark, so deal with it.

....

The aim was for Those Two Girls to be a full-time career when our youngest children started Prep. As it turns out, it happened a year ahead of schedule when, out of the blue, we were contacted by the founder of Australia's largest women's network, Mia Freedman.

For those outside Oz, Mia has been a media heavyweight since her early twenties when she became the youngest editor of *Cosmopolitan* magazine and is a name firmly entrenched in the zeitgeist for women since the 1990s. Turned out she'd been watching from afar and subsequently offered us a contract – $30,000 over four months to create content for her company. It was the first tap on the shoulder from a big gun, and the external validation we desperately needed to confirm we were on the right track ...

We then expanded into producing and hosting our own sell-out panel events for 400 to 500 women held in theatres, overhauled prestige showrooms, hotel ballrooms, industrial lofts and converted warehouses, netting upwards of $35,000 per night – which was not chump change eighteen months in. Our gut instinct was correct: women (like us) *did* want to witness female friendships played out in public forums; we were simply the conduit to see themselves reflected in our relationship.

It was 2016 and make no mistake: we were ON all the time. The green lights were pinging left, right and centre: we pitched client campaigns with integrated content (thanks to our shared PR and communications backgrounds), ditched all individual endeavours to focus on building together, and finally reached the point of enough financial stability to leave part-time corporate roles. We both did every. single. thing. And thank goodness our life stages were identical to mirror the time and energy required.

The next unexpected email would present a whole new direction. It was from Gemma Fordham, then head honcho at one of Australia's largest radio networks, Southern Cross Austereo, who had been watching our trajectory and range of projects with a plan in mind. She point-blank asked if we'd like our own weekend breakfast radio show.

Sidebar: Before going further, it's pertinent to understand how unusual this was; we hadn't sought out a broadcast career. The only randoms who scored radio contracts were former reality TV stars and the occasional retired athlete, and the typical flow was for presenters to start at a very young age and work their way through postings at regional stations, hoping to one day land a hotly contested job in a major metropolitan market. And the kicker? We were TWO WOMEN being asked to join the rare breed that is a female radio duo.

We point-blank replied with a resounding yes – our confidence yet again fuelled by our friendship, blind courage, and gumption.

In 2017 – the year we both turned thirty-seven – the next iteration of Those Two Girls began with a two-hour Saturday breakfast radio program.

In 2018, we accepted an offer to host a newly created national early breakfast show, live from 5 to 6 a.m. weekdays.

In 2019, our radio work expanded to include a three-hour local breakfast show – joining two male co-hosts – on Queensland's Gold Coast, bringing our tally to two shows and four hours of radio daily, Monday to Friday.

Beyond radio, we sat on stage in front of 2000-plus audiences and interviewed the likes of Sarah Jessica Parker, the Honourable Julie Bishop, Sarah Wilson and Leigh Sales.

But 2020 – the year we both turned forty – is where this story starts ...

ⓨ ⓨ ⓨ

As we looked down the barrel of a new decade, we began to question everything in our lives. From moments of overwhelm and frustration, to needing to reassess the stories and habits from our younger years, the entry into this new decade heralded changes, big and small.

Yet again we fell back on our instincts and asked the question: if we are feeling this way, surely we're not alone. Our podcast FORTY was born. It initially came from a selfish place: a perfect, legitimate ruse to seek out women with incredible tales to answer the curiosities we had. We figured every woman has a story to tell by the time she's forty. We were right.

Within ten weeks of launch, a publishing deal landed in our laps. Another green light.

The knowledge gleaned from our guests, and the critical thinking and self-assessment their words would give rise to, has been life-changing for us. Woven throughout this book are their lessons and wisdoms, along with a compendium of personal tales. Suffice to say, we are not subject matter experts on all things middle years, but our intention has always been to connect with people while being ourselves – and remains the utmost wish for this book.

Of course, it's a privilege to be living at a time in history where, as western women with a certain degree of comfort and education, we are in the fortunate position, and have the freedom, to express these thoughts, experiences, and conversations. We acknowledge these advantages and recognise our good fortune, always.

So, this is us, and the stories of how we came to know ourselves better.

This is forty.

Are you ready for this?

I've met some listless women in their forties and fifties ... who've taken the choice to do what others want them to do and put themselves last. They've become resentful and they've been sidelined. They've forgotten the joy, they've forgotten to participate in life, and not just live it for everybody else.

— Taryn Brumfitt

Carpe diem

Sarah

The death of my mother-in-law had a profound impact on me, although I didn't realise it at the time. It was only six months later when, at thirty-nine, I began to shake up the status quo of my life.

Ann was a kind and congenial lady – the type who did right by everyone, and everyone loved her for it. As an only child, she nursed both her father and mother through their elderly descent, and years later her husband, until he passed away after several strokes in his eighties.

When he died, Ann was in her seventies and had dreams of travel and cruises with her group of close girlfriends; several also widows. To all and sundry, this was an excellent idea – she was an active, vibrant member of her country community and, if not volunteering at the Salvo's store or the local historical society, you'd find her walking through her son's mango orchards or playing cards with her crew. She was so proud of not needing any pills at her advancing age, with excellent cholesterol levels, functioning knees and hips, and all her own teeth. Apart from a cancer scare resulting in a radical hysterectomy in her sixties, Ann was a poster child for a healthy geriatric gal. She set her mind to her remaining years being a time of freedom and exploration.

Then came the cruellest blow of all. Ann noticed a weakness in her speech. Her smile started to change. Her doctors initially put it down to old age, but she knew it was more. Eventually, after months of tests and specialist trips to rule out all other possibilities, came the diagnosis of motor neurone disease (MND). It's a death sentence that leaves a person trapped in their own body, unable to talk, walk, chew, swallow and, at the end, breathe. She died at eighty-three. A good innings, but an incredibly heartbreaking way to leave this Earth.

If anyone deserved to be graced the ultimate death of dying peacefully in their sleep at an old age after a life being kind and good to others, it was Ann. The unfairness subconsciously unleashed a kind of rage within me, although I only linked the two when writing this book.

Ann's death was the wake-up call I needed. You can spend your time being everything for everyone and putting others first and yet, when the time comes to do something for yourself, you may not ever get the chance.

I thought about my old-lady self. What would she wish she had changed if she could? Honestly, it was akin to an out-of-body experience. Blinkers were removed. What needed to change was crystal clear.

First went the job. In hindsight it's quite hilarious to recount, but Lise and I were offered a contract extension on a breakfast radio role we'd been doing for the previous year. It should have been a joyous moment – stability in the media is a rare thing. Instead, it involved me sobbing on the bed of a five-star hotel room with Lise slapping the mattress in frustration and yelling, 'WE CANNOT KEEP DOING THIS!' Quite the scene.

Needless to say, we declined the offer. Why?

For us, the hours were terrible – early and long – the job was 100-plus kilometres away from our homes, we were required to spend one or two nights away each week and our family life was suffering, our pay was not at all what people would assume and, overall, we were struggling. The cons far outweighed the pros – so, we made the call to leave with no regrets.

Next, came a major shift in my body image. Like many women my age and older, we grew up with the incredibly skewed perception that being thin coincided with being healthy and 'hot' thanks to nineties magazine covers celebrating Oprah's weight loss then criticising her weight gain, and Kate Moss mumbling through a durry informing an entire generation 'nothing tastes as good as skinny feels' (which, to be fair, I've read she regrets saying).

Throw in extra insecurity from my own bog-standard modelling years during the era of 'heroin chic' (the very definition of an oxymoron) and casting directors scrutinising my proportions or touching thighs (gasp!) and it was a match made in heaven for some quality skewed thoughts and hyper-awareness around how I looked in my twenties. For example, at 179 centimetres tall and a size ten, I was considered a big girl on the model books in a land of sizes six to eight, and regularly had to model plus-size label clothes on a catwalk. In the early 2000s, there was no one larger. No one. Back then, there were no other body types represented in the media. Praise be, this is no longer the case for young women. (On the upside, I often got to wear a wedding dress alongside the total spunk rat, faux grooms, given the super-slim gals couldn't fill the dresses out, so ... swings and roundabouts.)

At some point in my thirties – possibly after birthing daughters and praying they would not waste precious time and thoughts on such nonsense – this all became very tiring. It's exhausting narrowing your eyes at certain parts of your body and wishing they were different. I'd been 57 kilograms and running half-marathons, and 92 kilograms at full-term pregnancy and – spoiler alert – there was never a hint of a thigh gap.

Circling back to Ann, her MND diagnosis and decline was a

slap in the face to never whinge about my perfectly functioning, healthy body – or compare it to anyone else's – ever again. I could almost cry for those lost minutes, hours, days, weeks, and months of youth worrying about my figure, and taking on board other people's comments.

The other wake-up call around Ann's disease was nursing-home life – and seeing it from an adult perspective. Like many, I'd experienced it as a child when my grandmother Nano spent the last decade of her life bed-bound with Parkinson's disease, but it's different for kids, isn't it? Her nursing home felt a tad terrifying to our young eyes, and while my sisters and I loved Nano, memories of these visits merge with the smells of mashed potato and ammonia, sippy cups, wandering dementia patients, loud nurses, and bad daytime television.

But the way the oldies would look at us young'uns was something else: twinkly eyes with a glimmer of lost years and bygone pasts. I wish I'd said hello instead of feeling a teensy bit scared.

When your own life becomes closer to the finish line than the start, you view elderly people completely differently and think, 'If I'm lucky enough to grow old, what will that look like?'

Will I be the vibrant ninety-year-old with all my faculties, living independently, and hearing people exclaim whenever my age is revealed, 'Impossible! You can't be older than seventy!' I'll smile smugly and say, 'You have to use it or lose it', as I come in from pulling weeds to make a virtual reality call to my great-grandchildren from an embedded microchip. (This will be in the 2070s.)

Or will I be an old lady in the nursing home – white hair fanned out behind me in a recliner, feet with paper-thin skin and thickened toenails peeking out from under a crocheted blanket, jaw slack, eyes closed, *Play School* blaring, with my name never written in the visitor's book at front reception? Because, trust me, that happens, and it is heartbreaking.

I saw that lady every time I visited my father-in-law. (In fact, the saddest Christmas of my life was spending lunch there and seeing how many residents had no one with them. No one but the cheery, wonderful, paper crown- and tinsel-necklace-wearing aged care nurses to be the festive spirit – on their own Christmas Day – to lonely oldies.) Who was the old lady? No clue – except once upon a time, she was forty. Like me. Like you have been or will be. And hopefully she had a pretty rockin' life, chockablock full of good times and people so, when those eyes were closed, she was time-travelling back to them to ease the long days in the purgatory of prolonged and incapacitated old age.

This was another wake-up call: find the time between work and commutes and bills (generally running around like headless chooks) to make the memories that will become our olden days. No need for big or expensive. Throw a line in off a jetty. Fish and chips after a bike ride. A weekend by the ocean. A bushwalk to a view. A kitten under the Christmas tree. A play on opening night. An annual holiday. Anything at all with kindness, togetherness, or contentment. Treat people well, and hope they'll care and love you enough to sign a visitor's book one day.

Ann had lots of visitors.

She did right by everyone and perhaps that's one of the reasons she was able to maintain such grace and calm in the face of adversity. Her modus operandi was being a loyal, supportive, patient, helpful woman – even during her life's tumultuous times – but there was also an underlying grit and toughness. Ann was ten when the Second World War ended. Her rural childhood wasn't one of riches, and it involved the loss of her favourite uncle to suicide, plus her own loving father's alcohol demons – issues that weren't open for public discussion, such were the times. Those formative early experiences shaped her into the woman she became – someone interested in others, determined to see the best in people, and practiced in the mental discipline of active gratefulness long before it became a trend.

She nurtured her friendships. Her old canasta friends would come and hold the cards up and play for her, even towards the end. There were friends from primary school at her funeral. Chokes me up, even as I type.

And the final lesson from nursing-home life?

It's pretty handy if you can play the piano; immediate popularity in the geriatric set guaranteed. Ann could tickle the ivories with a multitude of rollicking tunes and, even though she'd lost her voice, one of the last videos I have is her playing 'Ain't She Sweet' a few months before she died. It's perfectly ironic – because my life's so much sweeter for having had her in it.

Evolution

Lise

Early in 2021, when Sarah and I first began thinking about this book, I fell hard and fast back into procrastination behaviours I thought I'd long shaken off. Any excuse not to start was a good one. Linen cupboards were reordered, bulk spag bol was cooked, my entire wardrobe purged and colour coordinated not once, but twice.

On one such afternoon, I decided to clean up the files on my old laptop, convinced it was a critical first step towards penning eighty thousand words. Amid old photos of the boys, renovation invoices, and downloaded immunisation records, I unearthed this little piece of angsty writing from 2018. I must have written it around the time Sarah and I began toying with the concept of a podcast about getting older. *FORTY* was a seed of an idea at that point, but I must have felt compelled to capture what I was feeling right then and there; to immortalise a moment in time.

Maybe it's kismet that our podcast about the middle years did come into being, because late-thirties Lise sure needed a good talking to from older, wiser women. Or perhaps it's kismet that I found this piece three years on, to appreciate just how far I've come since entering this decade.

I'll let you be the judge.

Journal entry by 38-year-old Lise – May 2018

I'm staring down the barrel of forty and I'm scared. Scared I'll become invisible. Terrified of being undesirable. It feels like I'm standing on the precipice of 'late-thirties' and 'over the hill', dancing right on that blasted edge, praying for a youth-and-peptide-infused jet pack to strap to my back and propel me onwards and upwards ... into what?

I don't know. Because I don't want to go backwards – really, I don't.

I like who I am at thirty-eight. I've survived the early, laborious years of raising my children, hit the pause button on my career more than twice, navigated ex-pat postings overseas, bought and sold homes, poured my heart and soul into establishing our family unit, supported my husband through a career change, figured out who I am as a mother, designed my own version of being a good wife. That was my thirties – sleep-challenged, maternal grit; a furious fusion of concern and anxiety, trial-and-error, family-focused endurance.

To be honest, I can barely remember my twenties, which is a good sign in my book. A blur of university life, jugs of Illusions, losing my driver's licence twice, half a decade of travelling, living and working abroad, an American male model boyfriend and carrying an inebriated Gisele Bündchen out of a Manhattan party.

I'm done with my second and third decades. Been there, done that, bought the t-shirt – Midori-soaked and arrowroot-stained.

And yet my fifth decade scares me senseless. I'm ashamed to admit my fear is borne of vanity. Like a right idiot, I have gone and indexed my worth to my appearance.

Because old habits die hard. I made a living as a fashion model on and off for twelve years. From the age of eighteen up until midway through my first pregnancy at twenty-nine, I was paid to look good and keep it tight. Then, I moved into 'commercial mum' territory, which suited me fine because I could eat normally and smile. Eventually, I got bored and disillusioned with the industry and hung up my flesh-coloured G-string. But make no mistake – years of viewing and assessing myself as a commodity has taken its toll.

My logical brain knows I am so much more than the shape of my body and the angles of my face. Still, I focus on both with a useless urgency, worrying, worrying about the day they will change, and I become unrecognisable to myself and others.

I look at my husband's ageing face and love it more with every line that appears around his eyes, every additional shake of the salt and pepper grinder atop his crown. The way his hands look rougher and yet softer at the same time; his gait – more solid, more dependable as the years go by.

There really is something quite magical about an ageing man. And yet I don't afford myself the same niceties. I just can't see myself through that same lens.

Instead, I've hit the panic button, dousing myself in coconut oil and performing nutcrackers at Pilates like a macadamia supplier on amphetamines.

I want to hear stories from other women. I want them to tell me it'll all be okay. I want someone to light a path for me, to show me a way, and then lots of other ways to navigate the decades ahead. I want other women, older women, to offer me new perspectives on ageing; to help me flip the script from anxiety to anticipation.

Present-day, 41-year-old Lise – 2021

First off, coconut oil made my shower tiles dangerously slippery, so I gave it the flick. Secondly, since turning forty I've done away with the punishing nutcracker drills and replaced them with weight training. I am now the proud owner of two callouses.

Maybe I'll start there, in this right of reply.

My attitude to exercise has dramatically shifted since entering my forties. My focus has moved outwards to inwards; from superficial to functional. I am suddenly acutely aware and in awe of what my body can do, and so the motivation to keep it moving, keep it agile, keep it strong, comes so much easier, and in a much healthier way than it did twenty years ago.

For a long time, I viewed exercise as a form of punishment – paying penance for something I'd eaten. My late teens, twenties and most of my thirties were spent reading nutritional panels, eliminating food groups from my diet, Tae Bo'ing and running in the nineties, spinning and Body Attacking in the noughties, getting closely acquainted with the cabbage soup diet, and buying over-the-counter amphetamines from a roadside chemist in Bangkok to lose a quick 5 kilograms before a big job in New York. And, hand on heart, I never even had an eating disorder. Never suffered from anorexia, bulimia or body dysmorphia.

No, I think my relationship with diet and exercise is probably quite familiar to most of you. Good foods, bad foods; good workouts, not-good-enough workouts. Before certain modelling jobs or ahead of show season, meals would become a transaction where I'd negotiate their terms and conditions with myself – 'I'll allow it, but it means no sugar whatsoever after 3 p.m., and you'll be going to that Pump class tonight!' A daily tug of war between 'you deserve this treat' and 'you did nothing to earn this reward'.

And even though it sounds exhausting, if I'm honest, I didn't really think much about it. I wouldn't even say I was tormented by any of it. It felt perfectly normal to me, keeping this mental ledger. Just part of my day, like brushing my teeth, or riding the subway. My peers employed similar techniques. I remember one particular summer in New York City, when one of my good friends, also a model, only ate Vietnamese rice-paper rolls and dehydrated pawpaw. Another colleague consumed turkey meat and a can of diet soft drink every single day over three weeks of Calvin Klein showings. We all shared low-calorie snack finds, like Cool Whip – a non-dairy imitation whipped cream. I can still rattle off the nutritional panel – 0 calories, 3 grams carbohydrates, 2 grams sugar, 1.5 grams fat. I have no clue what the hell was in it, but I ate it every day, out of the tub with a spoon.

With age and wisdom, I see just how disordered this behaviour was. Yet I've met so many women, from all walks of life, who've done the exact same thing at some point in their lives. Somehow, we normalised it, didn't we? Deprivation was desensitised. I spent so many years being unnecessarily strict on myself. The quiet self-flagellation, the unfounded self-reproach, the food fixation, although never extreme, was totally out of line.

Regardless of size – tall, short, slight, or fuller figured – it seems these kinds of thought patterns don't discriminate. I know I'm not alone here. But what I can say is this: I've found my footing in my forties. My approach is balanced and steeped in self-compassion.

I delight in the way movement makes me feel now, as opposed to seeing it as retribution for the quarter-pack of Aldi raspberry liquorice I put away last night. Now, I chase that feeling of accomplishment, the lightness of mind it delivers, the pride I feel when I see improvements in my strength and fitness.

As for food, just ask Sarah. Not a day goes by where I don't bellow, 'I've never been hungrier!' and then act on it within twenty minutes. Checks and balances and bargaining are things of the past. While I appreciate and uphold a sensible diet for myself and my family, I don't have time for neuroses. Now, my days are punctuated with gratifying food and drink moments – a warm bowl of porridge with lashings of honey, a vanilla latte sachet nicked from Sarah's top work drawer, ash brie and crackers with my husband Dane of an early evening. It'd be a shame not to, right?

In terms of how I look, well, I'm happy with how I'm tracking. I was never a great model, anyway – I was a good model who worked consistently, played it smart, and subsequently earned a decent living for a handful of years. But those days are done. I am more than my decade of modelling – to be defined by it or held hostage by a perceived pressure to 'maintain' it, would be idiotic. To be honest, I like my face better now. I've settled into its asymmetry. I like its angles.

Three years ago, I was scared, it's true. Frightened that crossing over into this fifth decade would mean I'd be dull and go unnoticed. But as new perspectives are offered to me, I'm learning that this is just the beginning.

How I wish I could credit the person who wrote this:

The reason society tells women they get less beautiful as they age is because women get more powerful as they age.

I remember furiously typing it into my phone. Let it sink in, as I did. Because what lies ahead is character and allure – a magnetism and *je ne sais quoi* reserved for the beguiling mature woman. For now,

I'm calmer, more self-assured. I know things. I have stories. And the pieces of who I am are falling into place, beautifully. This is how forty-one feels.

As I'd hoped back in 2018, the apprehension has given way to anticipation. Future-me, grown-me, the person I was always meant to be, is suddenly right here, staring back in the rear-view mirror of my compact SUV, at the traffic lights of a suburban intersection.

And yes, I am working towards seeing myself through the same lens, and with the same fondness in which I see my striking, ageing husband. I think he quite likes watching me grow older beside him, anyway. Because there really is something quite magical about an ageing woman.

I'm certain of it now.

How did you celebrate your fortieth birthday?

Lise

I was fifteen years old when Mum turned forty. I remember the evening clearly. She looked so glamorous – her hair in a long bob, a side-swept fringe, a mid-length pewter dress. The party was at home, mostly family and close friends. There was music and canapés, no caterers or anything outsourced. The women in our family had gathered in the kitchen the day before and the morning of, preparing the *amuse-bouche* ('mouth delights' – how good is the French language?), the crystal glasses, the napkins, and the outdoor area. Dad had worked in the yard the week prior and oversaw the procurement of all food and beverage supplies. The house was immaculate, the ambiance on point.

But what stood out to me most was that Mum wanted us kids there. There was no question in her mind that this celebration would include my sister and me. And for that reason, her milestone birthday became a family milestone – the first big, grown-up party we'd been properly invited to. So, when it came time for my fortieth in 2020, there was no doubt in my mind that I'd want my children with me.

My friends had been asking me for a while if I was going to go all out. A themed party, perhaps, or a big blowout at some inner-city hot spot. Maybe a destination event somewhere tropical. What about a girls' trip? A girls' lunch? Would I do something special, just Dane and me?

As a closeted introvert/introverted extrovert/social introvert/ ambivert/whatever the hell I am, the thought of an elaborate shindig with all eyes on me made me want to evict Rapunzel from her tower, move in, and give myself a two-blade to avoid any potential 'rescues'. The thought of Ubers, heels, event spaces, small talk, lots of people singing to me, speeches, outfits. No, no, no, and no.

It's not that I didn't want to celebrate the occasion. I absolutely did – I was so excited to turn forty. But in a strange turn of events, in late March of 2020, the world kind of shut down. And that was that.

My big milestone birthday became the most beautiful, low-key, comforting twenty-four hours in my own home, surrounded by my people. It was just the four of us – myself, Dane, and our children Remy and Max – and later Mum and Dad, who surprised me that afternoon with a veranda makeover – potted hydrangea working bee, anyone? (Baby Boomer parents go hard on a project, don't they?) – and a parental sleepover as the cherry on top.

The day started in dappled sunlight; much-cherished photos taken of me with my boys – the three of us still in our pyjamas. It ended by candlelight, eating triple-cream brie and quince paste, charcuterie, and marinated olives, and drinking exquisite French champagne – my children, my parents, and my husband by my side, raising our glasses to my fifth decade.

Just what this introverted extrovert ordered.

Sarah

Turning forty felt like a big deal. Teetering on the edge of the fifth decade, there was a definite demarcation between farewelling 'young Sarah' and welcoming 'middle-aged Sarah' and – the strangest thing of all – wanting to have a birthday party; wanting to be in the spotlight to mark this passage of time.

For many, it's not at all strange. There are plenty of folk who love a regular knees-up bash to celebrate the day they were born – and that's jolly good form *for them* – but it's not my jam. In fact, the last birthday party under my belt was my twenty-first. It was in the backyard of my family home, with the people who were important to me as I crossed the threshold from teen to young adult.

So, in 2020, the year of a global pandemic and entire city lockdowns, my birthdate somewhat miraculously scraped into limited restrictions of twenty additional people in one's own home; three days prior, that increased to forty – how serendipitous. The best part was the strict initial number forced me to curate a list of female friends who are incredibly dear to my heart, who had imprinted on me between childhood to age thirty-nine and left an impact. My invites landed on twenty women from various chapters of my life (some of whose thoughts and stories you'll read).

Just like my twenty-first, it was in the backyard of my family home, with the people important to me as I crossed the threshold to forty. It was my ultimate shindig: a beautifully set-up picnic under the stars, with cushions and rugs and flowers and fairy lights and nineties music, catered platters and delivered pizzas (no frills there!) and a giant coconut sponge cake with lemon curd icing decorated with nasturtiums. The lovely part was taking a moment to look at the wonderfully chaotic mix of people I'd collected since my teens ...

There were girlfriends from high school, who will forever be fourteen whenever my mind first flashes to their names; old friends from medical centres, where we worked together during uni years; a gaggle of hilarious, salt-of-the-earth women met during day-care drop-offs or in my own children's schoolyard; the best kind of grown-up friendships cemented in the grey-scapes of open-plan offices; former flatmates during single years; my lovely sister-in-law and sisters; and excellent ladies first brought into my life via the internet (including Lise!).

And then there were the two most important girls of all: my daughters, aged nine and seven. The funny thing is my initial thought when hosting the party was the kids probably shouldn't be there – it was to be a party for grown-ups with alcohol and fancy cheese boards. Then I checked myself – I was at my own mother's fortieth, a surprise party thrown by her friends, where she cried tears of happiness.

Then fourteen, I distinctly recall thinking forty was positively *ancient* – like a distant faraway land. No doubt my girls feel the same and given my youngest recently asked if I knew infamous 1880s bushranger Ned Kelly when I was a little girl, it's clear they are stuck in a time warp. So, they joined the fray, in party dresses and ribboned ponytails. Their very presence became a present, given neither of them had been born by my thirtieth birthday, and their subsequent addition to my life at thirty and thirty-two brought a happiness like none other, and continues to do so.

At some point in the night, I gave a little speech to the women who sat before me and explained how thankful I was to have accumulated them along the way. How, despite our lives moving into completely different phases and stages, they form the rich tapestry of my life. And how, if you're only as good as the company you keep, the faces I saw before me were the ultimate reflection of making excellent choices to accrue such a hotchpotch of legends.

While I held the floor for a couple of minutes, a friend snapped a candid crowd photo. In it are my girls, and they're seated near my feet, staring up at me with what can only be described as wonder and awe. A rare moment in time captured forever, where I can see their love shining through a lens, and I stop and think: if I'm not around for their own fortieth, they'll always remember mine – just like I remember my mother's – and the joy that was turning forty.

There was a three-week period where we opened up between COVID lockdowns, and in those three weeks, my two best girlfriends and me all had our fortieth birthdays. And all three of us had girls-only lunches at our homes, which is really indicative of who we are in the sense that we don't like men, we don't like going out of our homes, we only like each other, and we love getting drunk in the security of our own homes. And so, I had a caterer come in, I had this glorious bunch of women who are all in different life stages – some of them had kids who had just left home, and they were becoming empty-nesters, and others had just had their first baby – one of my girlfriends was sitting there drinking wine and pumping bottles of breast milk at the table. And eventually two people fell asleep, one of my friends with her face in her dinner. And – this is what I love about women getting older – this [other] friend, she's around fifty, so lots of good life experience, she doesn't fall asleep with her face in her dinner anymore, she went to the couch and procured a cushion, and then she leaned back in her chair and had it behind her head, and she just fell asleep like that. And I just thought, we know how to do it now that we're forty! And I thought, this is just a good, a good night.

— Sally Hepworth

I had a wonderful fortieth. I returned to where I went with my husband for our first date, when I was around twenty-nine/thirty, to Taronga Zoo. I'm really into the concept of Saturn Return. And so, for my birthday, with my two children in tow, we went back. That night we had a really fantastic dinner party with my closest friends, and we just laughed our heads off and had a really great time.

— Catriona Rowntree

It was a bit of a let-down, as I was in the midst of my cancer treatment. So, it was a non-event, so to speak. I think I was very much like, 'I'm happy to be here. Let's see where I go from here' – it was definitely not the fortieth I was expecting, but also, in a way, despite what was happening, it was still one full of a lot of gratitude.

— Sally Obermeder

[For] my fortieth I had a lunch for just girls. So, it ended up being forty girlfriends for a lunch and Jason, my husband. I wanted to do it during the day because I'm not very good at staying up late, and I get anxious being around people who've had too much to drink ... but then when I made a speech, I thought it would be really nice to mention the names – to acknowledge the names – of the babies that had been lost, because there was my good friend, Bec Sparrow ... she was there, she was actually pregnant with her second or third child, and we had bonded after we'd been introduced by mutual friends when she had a stillborn daughter, Georgie. And then I had another friend there whose daughter Maya had died at about age five months. And then I had another friend who had a stillborn called Katie. And so, I just thought it would be nice, because when you've lost a baby, as I did about

halfway through a pregnancy, sometimes it feels like that child is not real to anyone, but you ... So anyway, I thought it would be nice ... And, you know, you've got to be careful of rummaging around in other people's grief, as I've learned over the years, and afterwards all the women were just in the bathroom crying ... It was not my intention, but it was just like this absurd situation where I just made everyone cry at my birthday by trying to do this sort of thing. Anyway, it was a lovely, lovely lunch. I mean, it is love, it is life, right?

— Mia Freedman

I had a bunch of friends say, 'We've all chipped in. You can go anywhere you want to go – business class – New York, London, Paris – what do you want to do?' And I was like, I just want to go to a park and eat a sausage in bread. Because I spend so much time on airplanes, I just wanted to go to my local park and have the sausage in bread. And that's exactly what I ended up doing. And I was so happy.

— Taryn Brumfitt

For my fortieth birthday, I wanted to climb a mountain. So, my girlfriend at the time, we went to Bali to climb Mount Agung – that is probably the most dangerous mountain to climb because there's no safety. And so, I spent several hours, I think it was about an eight-hour experience, just terrified. I seriously thought I was going to die on my fortieth birthday, but it taught me a lot about myself: that I can just keep going and climb a mountain. I just wanted to conquer something. I think I just wanted to achieve something on my fortieth that I hadn't done before.

— Narelda Jacobs

My fortieth was only last year, so I had grand plans to have a celebration over in Europe. Obviously, that didn't happen [due to COVID-19]. My husband still made it special. He set up our apartment – he put 'Venice' in one corner. We had drinks in Venice, then went and had drinks in my office, in 'Paris', and 'Berlin'. So, I still went to Europe. It certainly wasn't as I had planned or hoped, but nothing in my life really is, so that was how I spent my fortieth. It was still a really, really great day.

— Lisa Cox

Well, as usual, I swung off a chandelier with a cocktail between my teeth. I think women need to celebrate every milestone because, when you have children, you take the burnt chop, you never get the window seat, you always put yourself last. You're tethered to the kitchen by your apron strings and your heartstrings . . . You're psychologically tethered. So, anytime you get to celebrate just being you, don't feel guilty. Women have a guilt gland. Our guilt glands throb all the time as mothers, we never think we're good enough. If we're working mothers, we think we should be at home doing creative things with Play-Doh. If we're stay-at-home mums, we think we should be out, striding the world stage with a couple of capital venture portfolios tucked up each sleeve. We just feel guilty all the time – and guilt is the gift that just keeps on giving. So never, ever feel guilty about celebrating your life and your sisterhood. Because my whole theme in life is that women are each other's human Wonderbras – uplifting, supportive, and making each other look bigger and better.

— Kathy Lette

I celebrated my fortieth in Hawaii and that's where my husband proposed. I totally stage managed it. I'd already designed the ring. I had about twenty friends and family in Hawaii for my fortieth, so it was just perfect that Darren was going to propose while we were there. He got to do that great thing – he went and asked my Mum and Dad, which is just the cutest – and then he got down on one knee in front of everyone, and we had my fortieth celebration that night. So, it was like a double celebration.

— Shelly Horton

I don't like my birthday, but not because of age, at all. I've got no problem with another trip around the sun. I've got no problem with getting older. I just don't like birthdays and I haven't ever since I was a kid. When I was forty, I would have had a ten-year-old and a five-year-old, so it probably was something like … I can't remember it!

— Paula Joye

The year of my fortieth birthday, I travelled to New York and trained with an amazing choreographer, Kira Armstrong. She's danced with some of the best, including Beyoncé, Jennifer Hudson, Lizzo. I hadn't danced in twenty-five years, so I booked seven rehearsals over two weeks to try and learn some fun and easy choreography that I could take back to Melbourne. I hired the Rising Queens – a beautiful, body-positive dance troupe – and they learned the choreography, too. Then we performed the dance at my fortieth birthday party in front of hundreds of my guests.

— Emmylou MacCarthy

I can't even remember. I've never been one for big birthday bashes and I particularly don't like that kind of attention that you get on your birthday when everyone sort of looks at you and they're like, 'So, happy birthday!' and you're like, 'Can you please stop, stop saying that'! So, I don't know. I probably had a dinner or something, but it was nothing big.

— Yumi Stynes

I probably celebrated it for about two years. It was like the festival of Ada! I always wanted to do something really big for my fortieth and I always wanted to go overseas, so we did. We went to Italy and to Greece with a whole lot of my friends. Hired a beautiful villa in Italy and it was just a really great time. I've always been excited about turning forty. And I'm not one of those people that hates talking about my age or was scared about the big 4-0. I was really excited about it. I just feel like a real grown-up now.

— Ada Nicodemou

I put together a wonderful dinner party for forty people on a rooftop in the middle of Sydney and it was sustainable. So, my poor friends had to be subjected to my whole zero-waste philosophy. I actually went and got a cut tuna carcass from the market, and we took out the cartilage from between all the bones and made this amazing tartare and put it in old tuna tins. And that was the entrée, and then made all these salads, and made everyone take the leftovers home. Everything was repurposed and reused. It was a fabulous night, actually – sustainable wine, zero sulphites. It was a really, really fun night.

— Sarah Wilson

We decided for our fortieth to have a B&S ball. Just down the road from our farm, there's this gorgeous little RSL shed, and we hired that out with all of our friends. We made an executive decision – there's no fancy food, there's no catering, there's no canapés. I think we did dumplings; we did sausage rolls; we did meat pies. We had five bottles of Bundy rum on the stage that you just went up and helped yourself with, and Coke bottles. Of course, we had wine and champagne and beer and all that stuff, but we didn't do anything elaborate. You had to dress in country and western and you had to dress a bit feral ... and everyone just killing themselves laughing as they walked in. I think it was just that wonderful step into this decade of going, we're not going to have airs and graces, pardon the French but we don't give a shit if people don't like the food, we're just going to have a cracker night with all of our friends. We put on really dodgy 1990, 1980s music – Madonna, Prince – and we just got really drunk and had the best night. I think I was still dancing on a wine barrel at about 3 a.m. in the morning. It was just a crackerjack night of relief, of excitement of ... you get back to a beautiful rawness, and you don't care, really. You're getting to that age in your life where, you know what makes you happy, you know who you want around you and you don't need the approval of anyone or anything.

— Gorgi Coghlan

Epiphanies

I wish I was less fearful of terrible things happening to me, because when terrible things did happen to me, I was brave enough to deal with them. I wish I knew that in every moment of horror and darkness in life, there would always be pinpricks of light. I probably lived with a bit of fear that something would happen to either my children or my parents, and I know now that terrible things do happen to people, and that you will be okay. Changed forever; but okay.

— Megan Daley

I hate camping

Lise

This is my sixth year of saying NO to camping. An assemblage of subpar experiences has led me to this point of total and utter roughin'-it-refusal.

Trip #1 – Neurum Creek, Woodford

Swayed by: The romanticism of our first family-of-four camping trip, campfires, cosy tent vibes, memories.

Reality: Five-month-old baby develops acute tonsillitis at 11 p.m. One minute I'm roasting a marshmallow and bouncing a healthy little ox on my knee, the next he has pus at the back of his throat. I lasted five hours of cluster feeding in three-degree temps before scooping him up, stepping over (read: ON) my husband, handballing the baby into the car, hurtling down the Bruce Highway straight into the GPs office, both of us in tears and needing prescription drugs. Amoxicillin for him, Valium for me.

Trip #2 – Gordon Country, Glengallan Creek

Swayed by: Upgrade to a friend's pop-top caravan, social camping with two other families, star gazing, kangaroos.

Reality: The region recorded its coldest temperatures in more than five years. My husband hadn't inventory checked the van's linen situation and all we had were threadbare Buzz Lightyear sheets, while the icy winds blew through the pop-top mesh. It was like a scene from the biographical survival drama *Alive* about the Uruguayan rugby team who crashed into the Andes Mountains and ended up turning to cannibalism to stay warm. The four of us had to sleep huddled together, wearing every article of clothing I'd packed, like miserable Michelin men. If you'd like another movie reference, I'm going to throw in *The Croods*. Remember the sleep pile? Dane on the bottom, the two boys sandwiched in the middle, me on top, cursing my decision to delegate the inventory check to Grug. At 4 a.m., when our youngest dropped his bottle because he couldn't feel his fingers, I once again tore down the freeway, baby in tow, landing on my parents' doorstep, too tired to drive the rest of the way home. Never saw a kangaroo but did name a star 'STUFF THIS'.

Trip #3 – Cotton Tree, Maroochydore

Swayed by: Swapping the bush for the beach, and winter for summer; the hire of a deluxe van.

Reality: Caravan comfort was exponentially better. What we didn't count on was the kids befriending a pack of rogues whose parents down the way spent the week boozing and passive-parenting, leaving me with five-year-old Sophia, seven-year-old Derek, plus our two boys on my lap asking me to read *Pig the Pug* for the 274th time in a stinking hot annex. Happy to help, love the spirit of communal camping (I don't – that's an outright lie), but Sophia ate all my cashews and strawberry wafers. There she was, every afternoon, showing up unannounced like a UTI, the rustling of the salty nut packet like Pavlov's bell. If that wasn't enough, I trod the path from our camp site to the dunnies that many times with all those small, sweaty, full-bladdered kids in tow, that it formed a channel. A deep trough of pain. Maroochydore is beautiful – if you can just get beyond the toot trench. Which I never did.

Trip #4 – Nature strip off the M1

I have no words other than Dane said the spot was serene and 'easily accessible'.

He was 50 per cent correct. He also said there was a waterhole for the kids and the dog to swim in. It was a dam full of thirteen black snakes.

I said many Hail Marys that night.

Now, half a decade on, the camping rules in our family go a little like this. I stay. They go. Their boys' trips have become a Dad-led utopia, where swags are rolled out, processed Cheerios in bread rolls are consumed morning, noon and night, Metallica is played on the drive, and no one really showers.

I watch on as they excitedly load motorbikes, coolers, barbecues and pillows into the box trailer and ute. I do my best to smuggle a tube of toothpaste and a zucchini into someone's knapsack. I dutifully ask for photographs of camp set-ups and tailwhips. And then I stand on our veranda, like a high priestess at her pulpit, waving them off, triumphantly.

I vehemently reject the idea that a mother's job is to 'fake love' everything her partner and children love. What does that teach them? That what Mum wants and likes doesn't really matter because what *we* like is what really counts. Thanks, but no. What my children and husband *need* will always be my true north. What they don't need is me hating on their camping fun just so I can tick the box and say I was there.

I am allowed to say, 'Guys, this isn't for me. Mummy's not the best version of herself when she has to wear double-pluggers in a communal shower.' They are with their father making memories, the same way they have made thousands of memories with me, and thousands more as a family unit. It is okay for me to sit some things out. It is okay for me to voice my likes and dislikes.

Tonight, we are off to see my son's school musical. On the weekend we rode our bikes for two hours along the esplanade after a game of touch footy in the sand. Last month we all went electric scootering along the river, stopping for Chinese on the way home. During the holidays I showed them how to play Dance Dance Revolution at the arcade. At Easter we went for night walks along the beach, sometimes close to midnight, just so it could be the four of us and the dog. Memories are made, with or without me pitching a tent.

So, this is a reminder that saying no to some things can make your yeses more considered, more meaningful, and extra special.

Mind the gap

Sarah

Oh, for years I wished for a thigh gap. It started in 1999 when I trotted off to a top modelling agency – with Kodak photos in hand – to join the fashion fray. Easy. I was tall, slim and white. Privilege! Surely it was only a matter of time before Cherry Ripe ads and Cayman Island photo shoots were in my future.

That was until the head agent looked me up and down, confirmed I was pretty, tall, slim and white, but immediately informed me I would need to have a thigh gap before being added to their books. Ouch!

For further impact, she then asked the model booker sitting beside me to stand up and show me her thigh gap, as a visual example. Honestly? I could have driven a MACK TRUCK through it. It was a thing of wonder. Light, quite literally, shone through her thighs. Magic. I nodded sagely, confirmed I would get one, and left.

....

Sidebar: Sarah Wills never did get a thigh gap. It was only after years of effort, she finally accepted her body was not designed to have a space between her legs for her food to fall through.

....

Fast forward to 2014, when Sarah Wills met Lise Carlaw.

Turns out Lise had a thigh gap *naturally*, and so modelled very successfully for many a year with that very agency. (One is reminded of the 'It's the fish that John West rejects that makes John West the

40

> I'm a lot kinder when I look in the mirror. In my twenties
> and thirties, it was always about 'do I fit in my jeans?' and
> 'I need to lose five kilos!' – just ratting on your body the whole
> time. Whereas I'm a lot nicer to my body, I'm a lot more
> grateful that it carries me around and has gotten me through
> so much.
>
> — *Sally Obermeder*

best' ad – Lise was THE BEST tuna, and I was the slightly dry one the trawlermen were like, 'Oh, well, not everyone's as picky as JW'.) Now, we're talking modelling in New York, Malaysia, France, Germany, Spain. Calvin Klein salon showings, Collette Dinnigan's fit-model, standing in for Adriana Lima in a Victoria's Secret light rehearsal. The real deal. I think she was also in *Vogue* in some obscure nation.

....

Lise's sidebar: It was *Harper's Bazaar*, Singapore, you silly binch.

....

The girl was a cracker, no doubt about it.

Anyhow, I was still in no-thigh-gap-recovery mode when Lise entered my life. I'm not going to lie – it still irritates me Lise never had to use 3B Action chafing cream during either of her pregnancies in a hot Queensland summer, but then she also never experienced the true joy of eating three Caramello Koalas every day for nine months and screaming 'IT IS FOR THE BABY AND I'M ON PROGESTERONE PESSARIES' at people because she was still modelling in her thirties. Sucks to be you, hot Lise.

But then came a revelatory turnaround. Hear me out.

One day at work, Lise said she had a weird globby thing on her

Your thighs touch, and that's fine ... I remember once wearing fishnet stockings and it was like I was wearing a cheese grater, my thighs rubbed together so much. So, get over that bit.

— *Shelly Horton*

shoulder. It felt like a little disc under the skin, and we had a bit of fun moving it around. Google said it was a 'Bible Cyst' and the best thing to do was, literally, smash a huge Bible on it till it exploded, dispersed, and was reabsorbed into the body. Given I was still channelling thigh-gap angst, smashing Lise with a Bible didn't sound unpleasant to me, but she decided against it and wanted to see a plastic surgeon. Vain.

Righto, so off she choofed to the doc who said it was, in fact, a lipoma – a slow-growing fatty lump usually detected in middle age – and he made a delicate cut and sliced it out then and there during the appointment. I can't tell you how annoyed I was that the only bit of extra fat on Lise was on her clavicle and able to be removed in ten minutes under local anaesthetic. (Also, did you know we are best friends?)

But then, Lise said, while there, she decided to ask him about something that bothered her A LOT. It was ... wait for it ... her bellybutton.

I kid you not. It certainly took me a moment to process ...

This total glamour, who'd made a motza modelling across the entire world, hated her 'outie' bellybutton so much she wanted to know if it could surgically be turned into an innie. In another irritating turn of events, the surgeon said her abs were so tight it would do more damage and he refused to operate. OH. MY. GOD.

Just to recap:

I have an innie and wanted a thigh gap.

Lise had a thigh gap and wanted an innie.

Deadset, we are one of those split love-heart necklaces girls give each other in primary school – together we are whole. It makes me a bit uncomfortable when Lise says she'd like to drink miso soup from my deep bellybutton, but when I mention getting my truck licence for a road trip through her thighs, it all evens out.

What's the moral of the story?

~~Even incredibly attractive folk fixate on parts of themselves.~~

~~If a surgeon can't fix it, move on.~~

Don't waste time loathing your body. No good will ever come of it. Also, do not threaten your friends with a Bible.

Discomfort zones

Lise

Ball sports have never really been my thing. I've never been
part of a ball sport team, which I blame my French parents for
entirely. As a first-gen immigrant child in Australia, oval balls were
suspiciously averted in favour of more solitary sporting pursuits like
tennis, pétanque, and teaching anglophiles how to emit the very
guttural French 'r'. (It's a sport – make no mistake about it: 'From
the *back of the throat* – repeat after me – the Disney rrrrrrrat is
called RRRRRRRRatatouille!') So, the irony is not lost on me, and
my entire family, that I ended up meeting, falling in love with and
marrying a professional NRL player.

Sidebar: Don't judge me. He's one of the decent ones. He owns a
pair of 'good thongs' and when he took me home to his parents
for the very first time, he insisted his mum cook her famous
rissoles, peas and chips. To this day, my mother-in-law Ann
reckons she died a million deaths when she realised this was
her son's idea of grade-A, bring-your-future-wife-to-meet-the-
parents cuisine. Case closed on normal husband justification.

Now, if you're anything like I was back then, you may be needing
a cheat sheet. NRL stands for rugby league, okay? It's the same sport.
Because I thought it was a whole other game, you know, like there's
rugby union with the cauliflower ears, AFL with the red ball and

Rebecca Judd, rugby league with the full-sleeve tatts, and then NRL, right? *Wrong*! I also once cheered for the opposing team in a semi-final. I'll never forget my father-in-law kindly applying pressure to my raised, celebratory arms, as he chuckle-hissed, 'We don't really do that in this section, Lise'. We were seated smack bang in the middle of Brisbane Broncos friends-and-family territory, while I chirped, 'But that was outstanding sportsmanship from the purple team, Gary! That Cameron Smith boy is quite good, isn't he! Has he been playing for long?'

So, when I birthed two sons, both built like their front-row father, I knew there'd be balls everywhere, quite literally.

My eldest boy has been playing AFL for a few seasons now. He loves it and we love watching him play. Does that mean I know what's going on when he's out on the field? Absolutely not. Do I reach my daily word count halfway through the first quarter, gasbagging with the other parents? One hundred per cent.

My husband has happily volunteered throughout the seasons – water carrier, coach's runner, flags, the works. Me? I've quartered Valencias under duress here and there, but I feel right at home washing twenty-five putrid jerseys in the privacy of my own laundry, so jumper duty is my nirvana. No prying eyes, nothing I can stuff up, just me and a two loads of pre-teen body odour. Bliss.

But that was then, and this is now. Since turning forty, I've challenged myself to step outside my comfort zones. Like, I might watch *The Living Room* one Friday night and then *Better Homes and Gardens* the following week. Sometimes I'll even buy Moccona instead of Nescafé. It's exhilarating.

So, you can imagine my smug satisfaction when I found myself volunteering as water carrier for my son's trial game the following week. This is what grown-up women do, Lise – they step up. Tired of being on the sidelines and letting others do the hard yards, this was me, strapping on an official team bib, and praying to the footy gods that I could hydrate those tweens like nobody's business. How hard could it be?

Game day. I'm wearing a lovely striped navy and white linen tee. Cool, breezy. A pair of Bonds shorts and my well-worn Nikes, hair in a high pony. It screams, UTILITARIAN SPORT CHIC. It says, 'I totally know the difference between a ruck rover and a fullback' – a magnificent gorilla, if you ask me.

I sidle up to the team manager to get an overview of what exactly water duty entails. He starts talking – fast. He mentions the fifty line (?) and says something about goals and poles, one flag waved versus two. My eyes glaze over and I realise I'm in way over my head. Say again, Darryl? I'm supposed to run out to those little bastards every time a goal is kicked? Why are they so thirsty? And I'm in charge of the backs. What about the fronts? Oh, there's no such thing as fronts? I knew that – was just testing you, Daz. And I need to know everyone's position, everyone's name, everyone's jersey number to run the correct water bottles out to the correct players?

Just as I'm about to suggest a cattle trough as the ultimate solution to this god-forsaken job, mother nature comes to my rescue, and the heavens open. An absolute torrential downpour. The kind that soaks my stripey linen tee in T-minus 45 seconds. Salvation, in the way of an unsolicited wet tee-shirt competition. I am saved.

Here's the thing. No one wants a forty-something-year-old woman frantically running up and down a footy field in a see-through top. It's a bit too Seminyak in suburbia; a bit too lamb-y for this mutton. The other footy mums come to the rescue. Tori immediately volunteers her sixteen-year-old as tribute. 'He'll do it. You clearly can't,' she declares. I suggest maybe swapping shirts with the kid, but I can tell he's not a huge Witchery fan.

Inside, I'm fist-pumping, grateful for the escape hatch, thankful I can return to the comfort of my chatty, coffee-fuelled sidelines. But my conscience tells me I'm bailing in spectacular fashion, all because I felt out of my depth running water out to my son and his teammates. What a cop out, Lise. What was I really worried about? Being laughed at for not knowing the game? YES. For not understanding the rules? YES. For feeling lesser-than in front of people who knew what they were doing? YES, YES, YES.

I must make good on my volunteering promise. But what other jobs need doing? The canteen lady just screamed at my friend Cindy for placing the frozen dim sims in the bottom, not the top tier of the steamer. But, frankly, if anyone can deal with dimmy fury, it's Cindy. She's got the cranky convenor covered.

Team manager Darryl strolls up and asks if I'd like to sit in the shade. I must give off strong sedentary vibes. 'Sure, I thought you'd never ask!' I reply, my resolve to step up to new challenges in this new decade easily extinguished. 'Great, Lise. I need you on scoreboard duty then.'

The world stops spinning, as Darryl punctuates his request with a slow-motion blink-and-smirk combo. What kind of ruse is this, Daz? Scoreboard duty?

That looming edifice in the top-right corner of the field that requires the poor soul in charge of it to climb a ladder in front of spectators, players and game officials, while manually hooking on giant number panels, ensuring the goals, behinds and totals are all correctly calculated? I mean, do I look like Russell Crowe in A Beautiful Mind? I don't even know what a behind is!

Darryl's wife, Ruth, rolls her eyes at her husband on my behalf, and jumps in to help me.

'We'll do it together so he can lay off me for the rest of the god-damn season. Don't ask me to do anything else, Darryl. GOT IT?', she calls out menacingly over her left shoulder, as we make our way across the grounds.

I'm madly googling 'AFL scoring' to try and make sense of the board's two rows and three columns. I know it's six points for a goal kicked between the two tallest white poles. Not too sure why the shorter poles on either side are there. Maybe it's for aesthetic balance? Why the hell haven't you been paying closer attention to your first-born and this ball game, you idiot!

Siren goes, and they're off. I'm praying it's a scoreless game. Of course, some little weasel kicks a goal almost immediately. It's a clear six-pointer. I rifle through the milk crate of heavy-duty plastic numbers. I yank out a six, climb the ladder, proudly hooking that digit up. Hands on hips – I've bloody done it. I'm on a roll now.

From across the field, Dim Sim Cindy is waving frantically at me. Has she copped more vitriol from The Tuckshop Banshee and needs to debrief? Mate, I'm an important game official now, it'll have to wait. Then I see Tori, doubled over in laughter, waving her index finger. Then from below me, Ruth starts shouting 'YOU WERE MEANT TO HOOK UP A 1, NOT A 6! THEY'VE SCORED ONE GOAL, SO THE 1 GOES IN THE FIRST COLUMN AND THE 6 IN THE TOTAL COLUMN! YOU'VE MADE LIKE WE'RE ON 36 POINTS! ABORT! ABORT!'

Cue circus clown music, as I desperately try to right my wrong. The kids on the field are looking up at the board, perplexed. The flag guys are laughing. I'm getting angry at my husband for being at work – how dare he – and at sport in general.

But I'm also laughing. And Ruth is laughing. Because this is all quite funny. Another overly adroit child kicks a goal through the shorter poles and calls out to me that it's worth one point. Okay, mate. You're a regular little condescending hero. One goal plus one behind equals seven points total. *Praise be*, I've got this, guys!

Ruth and I make it through the final quarter and are clapped off the field. I take it as a triumphant ovation, but perhaps the other parents are just glad we've finally stepped away from the scoreboard.

Moral of the story? You *can* teach an old dog new tricks. The big, scary thing you're often worried about never winds up being that scary, I can vouch for that. What I've realised is that when I'm outside my comfort zone, that's when I experience myself the most. Which is why I'll keep hurling myself out into the unknown, throughout this decade and the next, and the next again, because being uncomfortable can be great fun.

So, I've told team manager, Daz, that he can count on me for scoreboard duty this season. To be included in my rider: an assistant, a non-see-through shirt and a plate of top-tier dim sims, please.

Cemetery therapy

Sarah

Don't turn the page, hear me out: *I love cemeteries.*

Apparently, the official term is 'taphophile': someone who is interested in gravestones, cemeteries, and the art and history that accompanies them. Hi!

Perhaps it's worth disclosing I've dragged my husband to a mountaintop cemetery in Nice, done graveyard tours in Scotland, forced friends to detour through tiny alleys to spot old church-ground burials, made family pull over on country road trips to have a wander, and taken my own daughters on picnic lunches to them in my hometown until both my mum and husband said 'WHOA, YOU WEIRDO. STOP IT!'

It didn't help to have picked out my favourite grave – two sisters, Dolly and Little Jean, who died seven years apart in the early 1900s – and perched, eating sushi rolls, on a quasi-date with my girls and two spirit sisters. My thoughts were, how long since someone visited their graves? These two much-loved girls with the bird bath and dove carvings placed atop their joint resting place? It may as well be me and mine.

It was with joy and pride that I watched my girls find and fix flowers on graves. There's nothing scary or weird here. To me, they are sacred, beautiful, peaceful places for those gone before us – memories of lives and loves … and the ultimate place to visit if ever you find yourself at a fork in the road of life.

Every so often, the urge for a solitary sit in a cemetery will strike. It's usually always around a shift in pattern or life change, and it brings such a sense of calm and clarity.

We only have one life. Make good choices. We're a long time dead.

For example, at thirty-nine I briefly toyed with the idea of a third child when my two daughters were nine and six. And when I say 'briefly', I mean about six hours. The graveyard bug struck, so for two hours I wandered up and down rows of dearly departed, trying to figure out if I *truly* wanted another baby at forty or forty-one or forty-two? Did I want to go back to newborn life when I was now clear of sleepless nights? Did I want to risk a geriatric pregnancy, when my last one at thirty-three was hard enough? Did I want to be pushing sixty and still have a child at high school?

All of a sudden, the realisation dawned on me like a thunderbolt: I did not want a third child; I was simply grieving a chapter of my life that was over! Then I cried, felt the immense lightness that comes with making a decision, thanked the ghosts, and left.

Cemeteries are the ultimate destination for reminders about what is truly important: we should live the best life possible. Plus, sitting with spirits is a helluva lot cheaper than therapy.

Bosom buddies

Lise

I'm pretty sure I saw Jesus in December 2019. I remember there was a lot of white light; I was temporarily blinded, awestruck, speechless.

The world fell silent, and time stood still.

A wave crashed over my head, tossing me out of my reverie, as I dissolved into the kind of silent laughter that makes your obliques ache.

Jesus was, in fact, Sarah's left breast. Tata. Nork. Boob. Knocker. Bazooka. Jug.

There I was, underwater, howling with laughter, madly trying to make sense of why Sarah, *my Sarah*, was baring her bap in knee-deep surf on a crowded Gold Coast beach.

Six years of friendship and the most I've seen of Sarah's flesh is three inches above her right ankle.

Sarah is a lady. A maiden whose modesty and integrity are to be protected at all costs. Born in the wrong century, it's quite clear Sarah would have been a hybrid of Daphne and Eloise Bridgerton, while I, a fallen woman, would have rollicked my way through the brothels of 1800s London. Pulse points are where Sar-Sar draws the line when it comes to revealing herself to the world. And yet here she was, bust exposed for all to see.

Truth be told, I blame myself.

It was our last day of breakfast radio for the year. We'd finished an outside broadcast at Movie World, and Sarah had booked brunch at one of our favourite haunts to celebrate. It was there I proposed we wash off the year by running into the ocean. A cleansing ritual of sorts, to rid ourselves of the bad juju we'd accumulated throughout the year.

The weather was awful. Grey and overcast. Unusual for a December day in Queensland. We vowed to run up to our hotel room, change into our swimmers and march the half-block to the surf – no backing out. We were doing this.

To add to the excitement, we'd both been gifted a pair of togs ahead of the holiday season. Sarah had received a sun-safe floral one-piece, with a sporty zip from navel to neck. I'd opted for a neon orange number so high cut it was reminiscent of the insertion of my IUD, but hey, sun's out buns out.

Our hotel towels wrapped around us, we began the short walk to the ocean, mentally gearing up for our woo-woo wave clearing.

We dropped our white bath sheets on the sand and, with all the goosebumps and gumption we could muster, bolted towards the water. I dive under one wave, two waves. The icy water rendering me breathless but doing what I need it to do – shocking that year out of my system. I smile, knowing Sarah will be feeling what I'm feeling. I turn to find her, my Bridgerton bestie, and there she is, emerging from the sea foam, both hands grazing the sides of her head like Halle Berry in 007, head tilted back. She moves through the breaking waves, extending her frame into an upright stance – graceful, resplendent.

But something has gone horribly wrong.

The zip from her sensible bathers has betrayed her. The power of the ocean playing a cruel joke on my Sarah, unfastening her modesty suit in one fell swoop, the poor poppet oblivious to her plight.

Take me, wretched sea gods! Expose all of me, but not her! For the love of Poseidon, NOT HER!

Tata. Nork. Boob. Knocker. Bazooka. Jug.

I saw Jesus that day. It was a true Christmas miracle bestowed upon me, and the open-mouthed tourists on the foreshore that afternoon.

The image of Sarah slowly looking down, her gaze following my panicked, wagging index finger, and realising what had happened, will never, ever leave me. We laughed so hard, we cried. A white pointer sighting in the shallowest of waters. A spir-tit-ual encounter that I will cherish forever.

A state of undress

Sarah

At the start of summer school holidays, Lise and I decided to have a mini three-day getaway to the coast. We booked a three-bedroom apartment overlooking the ocean, piled the four kids into one car and drove down the freeway ready for fun in the sun (covered in SPF 50+, of course).

Her two boys in one room, my two girls in another, and Lise and I shared the main bedroom for the ultimate girls-night-in slumber party. It involved mismatched PJs, fluffy bed socks, eye mask, ear plugs, lavender balm, pillow spray, and a mouthguard to stop teeth-grinding – all of which was for Lise. I've known toddlers who've needed fewer sleep aids and wouldn't have been at all surprised if she asked me to gently pat her bum and sing 'Mr Sandman' to lull her off to the Land of Nod. All I can say is rolling over and seeing Lise all kitted up like that in bed ... well, Dane sure is a lucky man.

Anyway, this beach trip was different. At forty years old, I had a new outlook on life after my epiphanous year that was thirty-nine. In gratefulness to my working body, I'd decided to refocus exercise from solely running to several strength and high-impact training sessions a week under a local eight-week challenge run by a total powerhouse who was so passionate towards the women who fronted up and sweated and laughed under her watch. Burpees! Sprints! Plank taps! Goblet squats! Commandos! Boxing!

It changed so much inside my head, even more than my body.

Gone were the subconscious stories from my youth of being the tall uncoordinated girl who always stacked it in PE lessons at school (and always in front of my crush – *always*). Everything felt good. I'd never been stronger, more confident, and more aware that we have but one life to live.

On our first morning, we walked across the sand approaching the water. And instead of wearing the usual beach cover-up attire (rashie, sarong, huge hat, occasional board shots), I whipped out my secret weapon. And no, it wasn't a rogue breast – unlike the last time Lise and I were in the water together. It was a fuchsia pink bikini with a Brazilian cut bottom.

NEVER IN MY LIFE. It was so liberating – even though that pant style really does go up the jacksy at times – and guess what? Nothing happened. Nobody looked twice. Everybody was too busy going about their own beachy business to concern themselves with a married mother of two using her outer strength to not lose an eye putting the cheap beach umbrella up on a windy day, while simultaneously celebrating a newfound inner strength.

It unleashed some kind of bikini rampage, and I basically spent the entire weekend in a state of undress. The kids didn't bat an eyelid, and guess what? I asked my girls to take lots of photos of *me*. Too often, women are behind the lens, aren't we?

Furthermore, I made sure they captured a photo of Lise and me together in the hope they remember the power of female friendships by seeing how happy we were, how often we were in hysterics, and how comfortable we were in our skin together in the middle years of life.

Mummy loves you, you sexist jerk

Lise

It's 4.08 p.m., my boys have been home all of seven minutes, and I've just called my seven-year-old a sexist jerk.

Here's the thing: I don't regret it.

Was it age-appropriate and unnecessarily harsh? Probably not, and absolutely.

But I had a point to make. I *have* a point to make.

A few days each week, my two sons catch the school bus to their respective institutions about thirty minutes away. The bus ride into town is a charming cacophony of fart competitions and TikTok videos, set to the aerosolised soundtrack of Lynx Africa blasting into teenage armpits. It's boy-heaven in there. My two alight at the same stop, parting ways with little more than a brotherly grunt. The little one walks 11 metres to his campus while the older one takes twelve strides west to his, the terrain flat and idyllic, lined with cherry blossoms and the odd crucified Jesus.

The details here are important. My children are not enduring a daily cross-continent expedition à la Burke and Wills. At worst, the tween may forget to charge his Samsung A11, resulting in a missed backseat music sesh with 'da boiz', or the little one will have snapped his go card in half from commuter boredom, leading to an accusation of fare evasion by Tim the disgruntled busso.

It should also be noted that out of the ten possible journeys to and from school each week, my husband and I will facilitate sixty per cent of them. Wednesday, for example, having finished work a little earlier than expected, I put in a call to Annette on junior campus and 'Front Desk Liz' from middle school and arranged a sneaky 2 p.m. surprise pick-up. As soon as Max, my youngest, locked eyes with me from across the quad, I knew I'd come through with the maternal equivalent of a division one Lotto win – I'd spared my child from a forty-minute Ash Wednesday Liturgy in the multi-purpose hall. My eldest was equally chuffed, narrowly dodging a Mr Briden-shaped bullet after realising he'd forgotten his saxophone for sixth-period band rehearsal. Big Mama is a walking Power Ball, babies, and don't you forget it!

But forget it they did. Or at least the seven-year-old did.

Which brings me to today. The front door swings open. I am greeted by a peppy man-child who seems mildly buzzed from some contraband Wizz Fizz. I welcome the chemical positivity for now, and bowl him a Granny Smith to counter the effects of Preservative 220. But Max, the cherubic baby of the family, looks downright miserable. Eyes downcast, pouty, stompy. Not his usual mojo.

'What's wrong, honey?', I ask, dutifully.

And then he delivers the words: '*Why don't you ever pick us up? You're home so you could have picked us up. I don't like walking up to the house. You're not even at work.*'

Remember those neon glow sticks at raves back in the early 2000s? Well, all of a sudden, I'm one of those – some rabid lunatic who's dropped an E has just cracked me a little too hard, heck, he's bitten down on me, and now I'm glowing hard, flaring up, spewing out my toxic phosphorescence.

Before I know it, the hives start forming on my neck-and-dec as the words tumble out of me: '*I've been up since 2.50 a.m.; at work all day; interviewed a senator; home in time to put dinner on, to make your beds, to do your laundry, to reset the house before the arrival of Little*

*Lords Fauntleroy; all while my eyeballs are hanging out of my head;
to submit your Rugby League club registration and respond to some
random junior coach about what nickname you'd like to choose (FYI,
I've gone with 'Beelzebub'); to locate your left-handed scissors because
god forbid you should experience the hell that is non-ergonomic cutting
in tomorrow's art class!*

Breathe.

The tirade continues … and this time, I can feel the beginnings
of my feminist flag flapping out of my Bonds briefs. This is going to
be good.

'You would NEVER *say that to your father! Why? I'll tell you why!
Because he's a man and you wouldn't dare suggest that a man should
sacrifice more – more, please-Sir-I'd-like some-*MORE *– for his children!
No, that kind of torture is reserved exclusively for mothers – ooh-ee,
aren't we lucky!*

Breathe.

The flag is flying at solar-plexus level now. It's time to bring in the
career chat.

*'Is it because he wears a uniform, and I don't? Would you like me to
wear a uniform to my mid-dawn breakfast show? Would that stop you
from asking me to drive the twenty-three metres from bus stop to door
stoop? Would that* VAL-I-DATE, *in your eyes, what I do from Monday
to Friday? I'll just jump on eBay and bid my way to a maid costume,
shall I?*

*'Well, the jig is up, junior! How convenient that you've forgotten
yesterday's early mark! Shall I burn dinner, gather the ash from the
oven and recreate Father Joseph's sermon for you? I have a better idea.
How about you catch the bus ten times next week so you can feel the
full brunt of what it could actually be like …*

*'*YOU SEXIST JERK!*'*

At this point, my husband is staring at me, mouth agape.

Hesitantly, warmly, in fact, he says, 'Come on, settle down a little, Lise.'

Remember Billy Blanks, American martial artist and founder of Tae Bo? I could have roundhouse kicked my husband in the thorax at that point.

Instead, I collected myself, somewhat, and through clenched teeth, I hissed my final coup de grâce: *'To think I even had a Milo and a Ferrero Rocher ready and waiting for you.'*

And with that, I turned on my heels, ordering my husband to workshop what had just happened with his son so he could hear and understand it from a man, because obviously we'd created some kind of misogynistic wretch who wasn't fluent in Uterus.

Look, it wasn't my finest parenting moment, I'll admit. The kid hit a nerve on a day where I was feeling the overwhelm of being a working mother in her forties. What it did, though, was start an honest conversation between us about why my feelings had been hurt and why I'd said what I'd said; why I felt that the demands on Dad sometimes felt wildly different to the demands made of Mum.

My sweet boy is not a sexist, entitled jerk. He is the opposite of that. I hope, in part, because I've let him in on the inner workings of my mind. That day Max learned what sexist means and why being that way is not okay and not fair. That day my husband learned that the weight of invisible expectations can bear heavily on my shoulders. That day I learned I should favour chamomile tea over coffee before the kids come home from school. And that using my voice and being vulnerable in front of my boys is not the end of the world.

You'll be pleased to know that dinner was neither burned, nor applied to my kids' and husband's forehead in the shape of a cross.

Thanks be to God.

Womanhood

This time of our lives can be so empowering if we are willing to take charge of it, and not feel this sense of 'I'm at the mercy of my hormones'. Not 'I'm going to fight them', but 'I'm going to work with them, I'm going to acknowledge them and own what I need to do so I can show up'.

— Kemi Nekvapil

Coming up for air

Lise

When my kids were little, life felt like a quagmire of sleeplessness, regimented routine, and noise. I've said it once and I'll say it again – I didn't enjoy the early years of parenting and really struggled with the intensity of it. I held myself to impossibly high standards set by infant sleep experts and French family who couldn't handle the sight of a filthy highchair, or a *bébé* who didn't wear leather booties 24/7. (It's a Francophile thing, the baby/shoe thing. Look it up.)

My husband and I had our first child when we were living in France. We were both twenty-eight, and it made sense to start breeding during our expatriate years. Dane was rounding out his NRL career in Australia and, like a lot of athletes looking to ease into semi-retirement, he was snapped up by the European Super League – the professional rugby league competition in the Northern Hemisphere.

While most clubs are scattered across northern England in dull places like Liverpool, Leeds and Wigan, we struck expat gold when Dane signed with the Catalans Dragons – the only team based in the south of France, in the idyllic seaside town of Perpignan. 'Perps', as we affectionately called it (find me an Aussie who won't sniff out the diminutive form of any given word), is a utopia of vineyards, colourful beach clubs and quaint village squares, straddling the French and Spanish borders. We spent our days training (Dane) and eating Nutella crepes by the seashore (me).

After enjoying a year of travelling through Europe as newlyweds, riding Vespas, getting drunk in cobblestoned streets and stuffing our faces with foie gras, we decided to start our family. Reality set in when my due date collided with the Super League preliminary finals. With Dane's team in the play-offs, we were told in no uncertain terms by club management that no baby would get in the way of their Grand Final chances. *Merde*. That's French for 'shit'. It's par for the course as a professional footballer that chasing pigskin takes precedence over most things, but also, *merde, merde, merde*.

It would mean being alone – no mother, no sister, no best friends by my side – staring down the barrel of birthing a 112-kilogram front-rower's spawn. *Au revoir*, vagina. 'Twas nice knowing you. Long story short, we pleaded with my obstetrician to induce me two days before Dane was due to fly out and play in St Helens. The pressure to perform felt greater than the nine-pound unborn baby that was doing the Pachanga on my perineum. Remy was born on 9 September 2009 at 9.05 a.m., and Dane flew out the very next day. We had one night together as a family of three, and then I was all by myself in a French maternity ward with no wi-fi to Skype family back home. I remember standing beside the hospital crib, engorged norks out, wearing a giant adult nappy, crying.

I became a long-stay roomie at the *Clinique Notre Dame d'Espérance*, bunkering down until Dane's return, with occasional visits from my expat girlfriends and curious French midwives who wanted to meet the only breastfeeding mum on the ward. (True story. At the time, the trend in France was very much skewed towards bottle feeding, and most mums on my floor had requested tablets to dry up their milk. I was the only one who was keen to give it a crack.)

Now I look back on it all, it was pretty dismal. Tough on me, tough on Dane. We were apart for five days. Or was it seven. I can't remember. Nor can I remember most of that first year if I'm honest.

There was a particular low point where I became a literal stage five clinger, clutching at Dane's ankles begging him not to leave, when, just three months later, he was back on a flight to England for six weeks of pre-season training. I remember howling through the computer screen to one of my girlfriends, Remy on my breast, alone in our house, wondering how the hell I was going to get through the next few hours, let alone days. But we survived, and it made me spectacularly independent and resilient when it comes to pulling my big girl pants on. Unsurprisingly, we didn't last long in that set-up and decided to farewell France when Remy turned one.

Once back in Brisbane, we lived with my in-laws for three months, our belongings in a shipping container somewhere in the middle of the Southern Ocean. I was always tired, living out of suitcases, trying to make sense of this new life we'd found ourselves living. Eventually, we moved into our own place, and soon after I suffered a late miscarriage that would take the wind right out of me.

I was three months' pregnant, a lovely little belly proudly poking above my waistband. I'd been booked in for the standard twelve-week scan, a 7 a.m. appointment that meant Dane could stay home with Remy while I zipped out. It wasn't my first rodeo, after all. I was fine to go it alone.

The look on the sonographer's face as she glided the handheld probe over my tummy made my neck feel prickly and hot, but as I lay on my back staring at my swollen middle, I convinced myself everything was fine – of course it was! But it wasn't. The foetus hadn't progressed. It's what's called a missed miscarriage, where your body continues to develop as if the pregnancy is perfectly normal even when it's not. It's the cruellest form of gaslighting.

I was blindsided and felt so, so stupid. The sonographer gave me some time alone, apologising quietly on a loop as she walked out the door. I called my sister and wept. I was sitting half-naked in some weird little cubicle, my vision blurry, my choked sobs interrupted by my rational brain telling me I'd be fine, that women suffer far greater losses every single day. My sister begged me not to get behind the wheel, but I needed something concrete to focus on, and wanted to get home to Dane.

The following week was a blur. I was given the option of a D&C, a procedure to clear the uterine lining after a miscarriage, or I could miscarry at home, naturally. I was told that my body would eventually expel the mass in my womb. I have no idea why I didn't choose to go under and just be done with it. Maybe that would have been easier. Instead, at fourteen weeks along (but not – what a mind bend), the tightening spasms began, in the dark of our bedroom. I remember the flicker of the television sparking beneath our bedroom door. I had asked to be alone, knowing Dane was just a few feet away.

Several hours later I felt something slide between my legs. I ran to the toilet – so scared, so scared – and called out to Dane. I could barely look at what had fallen from me. Dane took over. I'm not sure what he did. I can't remember. I'm ashamed to admit all of this, as if somehow my inability to face it all makes me a heartless mother. But no one had prepared me for any of it – what I could expect to see, what I should do with 'it', what 'it' even was. Just a slippery sac of organ-like tissue? Is that what I glimpsed, before squeezing my eyes shut and holding my breath?

Young women reading this, do me a favour. Please ask if you need to. Put your hand up and ask the older, wiser women in your circle what you need to know. You are owed details and information if you want them. Why the doctors never stepped me through the process, even an abridged version, I'll never quite understand. Perhaps they did. Perhaps I was too busy staring out at the fig tree one of the nurses had pointed at, telling me some parents like to bury 'whatever passes' under it. We offer that, should you wish. Here's a pamphlet. Um, sorry, what am I burying? Won't it just be blood? Again, blur.

The fact is, I got through it. It was a pivotal, primal moment in my life as a woman. An education in the fragility of life and the magnificence and intuition of the human body. Something that will bind Dane and I together, silently. Dane never wanted me to go through anything like that again. Nor did I. My insomnia came back, my complexion was drawn and grey, and I was terrified of falling pregnant and miscarrying again, and again, and again.

Miscarriage is part and parcel of being a reproducing woman. These things happen to so many of us. Does that make it any easier, knowing our sisters, mothers, friends and colleagues have walked a similar path? Absolutely not. It's your experience alone to carry. Some women will remember the exact dates, or plant shrubs to remember the babies that never made it earthside. Maybe they'll opt for the fig tree package. Everyone is different. For me, despite a sadness I still carry with me, and tears that fall each time I recount the story, I don't associate the experience with a little person that should be here with us today. For me, I can rationalise it as a cluster of cells and tissue that just never grew. I had another miscarriage after that, at eight weeks. I cried, again, but it's just part of life, isn't it?

In a serendipitous twist of fate, turns out my woeful progesterone deficiency (the culprit of my multiple miscarriages) is how I found my way to Sarah. Soon after meeting online, she and I swapped stories and connected the many dots of friends we had in common, and times and places we should have met but hadn't.

We were both pregnant during our Facebook Messenger courtship of 2013, and it was over the course of a late-night chat we discovered we both had paltry progesterone and were seeing the same specialist. I commiserated with Sarah over her pessary treatment, while I graduated to weekly jabs in the bum to keep Max's hold on my uterus firm and steady. When I finally held my second-born in my arms, I exhaled deeply. Sure, the scar tissue in my right butt cheek had hit pork crackling status from nine months of needles, but the little blighter held on strong, with the grip strength of a ninja warrior on the salmon ladder. We made it, kiddo.

My story is an ordinary one. Probably not dissimilar to yours, or someone you know. It makes up the many twists and turns of jumping on the reproduction rollercoaster. But the baby making and birthing part is just the beginning of the ride, really. What isn't spoken about enough, in my opinion, is matrescence – the 'making of the mother', where you're thriving one minute and distressed the next. It's a confusing clash of emotions that colours the many years beyond labour. The transition from woman to mother is monumental and, in my case, it was lengthy – I would say a decade long.

Why don't women talk about this more? Why didn't someone draw my attention to that scene in *Ace Ventura: Pet Detective*, where Jim Carrey is birthed out of a robotic rhino, and say, 'See this, Lise? This is how it will feel becoming a mother. It'll be a long and arduous process, equal parts beautiful and confronting. Eventually, like Jim, you'll come through and be able to breathe.'

My sister was one of those allies who gave it to me straight. She gave me permission to let it all out and made me feel understood when I called my two-year-old an asshole. The truth is my thirties were a pull and push of wanting to breathe my boys in but craving physical and emotional space. I walked the line between elation and exhaustion often. I'm not talking about postnatal depression. That was never my reality. But there's a grey area between that clinical condition and the mum on the Nurofen ad who looks put together, rested and genuinely thrilled to be dealing with her congested toddler. The experience of early motherhood is not good or bad, it's both good and bad. At least that's very much how I felt.

But here's where it gets good – and I'm writing this piece for all the women who may be deep in the trenches of matrescence. Hang in there, girls. Because when you make it to the other side, there is delight.

You see, I've finally entered the golden age of parenting. This is the age where the boys are old enough to be independent, but still young enough to love Dane and me like we're demigods. They can walk to the IGA by themselves, but still want me to massage eucalyptus rub into their pulse points before bed. It's precious, rewarding and the very best fun. Now, at forty-one, I've finally arrived at this destination, and I've never been more certain of who I am as a mother.

And here's the kicker. I'm not tired anymore. I know, it's taken me that long – my kids are eleven and seven (throw in revolting breakfast radio hours that most certainly stunted my road to enlightenment) – but that fog of stress, anxiety, and burdensome responsibility has finally lifted, and through the brume is delight. Because delight can only re-enter your life when you've kicked fatigue to the kerb. With older kids and better work hours comes the gift of time. I now have time to delight in the little things.

In my forties, I'm noticing just how many moments of joy are present in my day. I've grown to recognise how essential it is to acknowledge and embrace those moments that fill you with delight.

I love that I've arrived at a place in my life where my head is out of the proverbial rhino's rump, and I can savour all the juicy little moments life has to offer.

So, I took to social media with these musings:

What do you delight in?

What are the little things in life, those magical moments that bring you joy and make you feel wonderful? For me it's things like:

- pulling on trackie pants in winter
- a glass of wine on the veranda with my mother-in-law
- decluttering shows
- dippy egg night with the boys
- riding electric scooters along the esplanade
- watching our dog play on the beach
- singing in the car
- sharing a bucket of prawns with Dane
- eating Darrell Lea choc-raspberry balls alone in the car ride home from getting the groceries
- diving under a wave
- a whole day stretched out in front of me with no plans
- goat's cheese and apricot jam toasties
- family conversations at the dinner table
- being tucked up in bed
- Dane wearing trackie pants (it happens once or twice a year. Like a partial lunar eclipse or a blood moon)
- motorbike rides to inner-city laneways
- long runs alone
- pizza night with my parents
- uninterrupted phone calls with my sister once a week.
- Over to you!

~ Lise

It seems many of you have hit the Delight Milestone, too. Here's what's enchanting you in your forties:

- lying in bed reading a book
- spending time laughing with friends about life
- leftovers in the fridge
- a swim in the ocean
- settling into a great Netflix series
- going out for breakfast
- embracing sentimentality
- the first spoonful out of the peanut butter jar
- electric blankets
- getting ready to go out
- that first sip of coffee
- fireplaces
- folding sheets (Um ... I have so many questions)
- designer pyjamas
- hugs from teenagers
- cups of tea on the veranda watching the storm roll in
- afternoon quickies before the school bus arrives
- a great cheese platter
- impromptu singing
- fresh sheets on the bed
- Sunday sleep-ins
- swimming late at night when the kids are in bed
- well-made leather boots
- clinking champagne glasses with good friends
- alone time in the morning before anyone else is awake
- making a complex curry with all the ingredients
- foreign movies
- Sunday baths
- going to bed early a few nights per week

- friendly service
- slipping on a dressing gown after a hot shower
- sunrise dog walks
- reminiscing about nights out fifteen years ago
- removal of bra at the end of the day.

So, while the young fillies around us may have youth on their side, collagen in spades, perky glutes, and enviable upper-breast volume, what we mares have is far richer. We have the gift of time, the gift of paying attention, the gift of noticing and soaking up the slivers of bliss present in our everyday. There is such delight to be found in lingering, loafing, lazing, lounging, meandering, puttering and moseying – a joy reserved for our middle years now our heads are finally above water.

Midlife motherhood

Lise and Sarah

Geriatric pregnancy – ugh. It's an abrasive term, but science says our weeny little ova start to lose their punch as we edge closer to midlife, and the statistics don't lie when it comes to possible difficulties and risks for women who have kids after thirty-five years of age. Sure, biologically speaking the preference would be to start birthing babies in our teenage years, when eggs are ripe and ready, and while this was tickety-boo in our grandmothers' generation, times have changed.

Sidebar: My grandmother had her first child at eighteen, and her first grandchild at thirty-eight. Lise's grandmother became one at forty.

Many, many women are simply not in a position to have a child until at least their mid thirties – and for myriad reasons, all of which are no one's business but their own. There are several mothers in our circle who had babies in their late thirties or forties – and their stories are so vastly different.

Andy's story
Sarah

At twenty-one, one of my oldest friends from school days, Andy, was *finally* diagnosed with endometriosis after suffering debilitating menstrual cycles for years. First whammy was the poor thing got her period at ten and was sick – migraines, cramps and excessive bleeding – every month from very early on. By her recall, three out of every four weeks involved ongoing pain. Look up a medical explanation of severe endo and her name should be there, then came polycystic ovaries to boot. During Andy's first laparoscopy, the gynaecologist removed not only the thickened tissue in her uterus, but also a substantial amount adhered to her bowel. In other words, she was riddled with it and, while the initial diagnosis delivered a major dose of relief, it also came with a hefty dose of doctor's advice to have a baby as soon as possible before it further impacted her fertility.

How easy to say; how difficult to do. Like many women, Andy simply wanted to have a baby with the love of her life ... but had had to spend more than a decade wading through the waters of dating in her twenties and thirties.

'There's only so many things you can speed up,' Andy said. 'As I got older, the knowledge I may not be able to have children had a significant impact on the type of man I wanted to be with – someone who would be okay with *not* having a child, and who would feel fulfilled sharing a life together as a couple only.'

Said man entered, stage left, when Andy was thirty-four, and she married the lovely fellow at thirty-seven.

Next, was the wait to have a baby. In conjunction with existing fertility issues, scar tissue from three laparoscopies, plus throw in all the potential complications around advanced maternal age and Andy never needed a reality check as to the likelihood of motherhood. Quite simply, the years of being told how minuscule her chances were of conceiving naturally meant she had been slowly grieving the fact a child may not be in her future and had looked firmly down the lens of a life sans children.

On how she handled the years of friends around her having babies while managing her own yearning: 'I was determined not to let other people having babies get in the way of my happiness for those babies. At the end of the day, I didn't want anyone else's, I wanted my own.'

Her lady parts had already been poked and prodded so much – with the scars to prove it – plus having worked as an IVF nurse meant she knew the uphill battle to be faced. She'd counselled and nursed so many women in similar scenarios to herself, had seen how addictive IVF could be in the desperation to have a child and the strain it put on relationships. Andy decided it wasn't the right path for her; instead, she set a firm timeline: if she hadn't fallen pregnant naturally by forty, she would move on with life, with the full support of her husband.

For two and half years, they tried to no avail.

They bought an SUV – purely because it was a good deal, but she can remember thinking, 'I've got the family car, now I just need a baby to go in it'.

Then – seemingly against all odds – at thirty-nine, Andy fell pregnant.

'It wasn't a jump up and down moment, it was pure shock,' she recalled:

It took months until it felt real. At my twelve-week ultrasound appointment, my obstetrician left the room and I turned to my husband in disbelief and said, 'There really is something in there!' Then at thirteen weeks, I bled overnight and was convinced my one chance at becoming a mum was all over – and wasn't even surprised given all the risks being pregnant at my age, but the baby stayed.

Twenty weeks was a turning point for me. I spent an entire weekend in tears realising I was actually going to have a baby, but then the worry and panic kicked in. Am I too old? Will the baby come early? Will he or she be in neonatal intensive care for months? I'll never make it to full-term, and so on. It was completely overwhelming.

I felt I needed to be mentally prepared for any potential issues, so we had recommended tests and genetic screening to make sure our ducks were in a row in case of complications, plus I diligently monitored the baby's movements – one of my good friends Heidi lost her daughter at forty-one weeks' gestation, I knew I didn't want to risk going past forty weeks.

At forty, Andy had a baby girl – a blinding light of pure joy amid the global upheaval of 2020. While the pregnancy was blissful ('I'd never felt healthier in my life'), the birth was a hectic affair. Bub's growth had slowed in-utero and she was a footling breech, refusing to turn. Andy's no-nonsense approach meant she readily agreed with her doctor to have a caesarean at thirty-seven weeks. Not only was her daughter's cord wrapped around her neck twice, but there was clear visual evidence the placenta had started to fail in the final weeks of pregnancy. It was sent to the lab for analysis, which confirmed 'placenta accreta' – a serious condition that occurs when the placenta grows too deeply in the uterine wall, and typically detaches after birth causing severe blood loss, often requiring an immediate and complete hysterectomy. It's an increased risk for pregnant women over thirty-five, as is surgery that leaves scarring on the inside of the uterus. Given Andy had three laparoscopies at age twenty, twenty-four and thirty-two, the latter was a possibility.

Over a cuppa, I asked if she ever felt judged for being an older mother.

'No, actually. Even though everyone in the mother's group I joined was younger, I never felt out of place; a baby is a great leveller, whether you're twenty-five or forty-five,' she said. 'Interestingly, my

In all honesty, I think I'm a really good example of a late bloomer and I think if anyone else is panicking or feeling uncomfortable heading into their forties, I'm here to tell you just don't be. Everything big and huge and life-changing actually happened to me after forty, and indeed after fifty. So I think I'm a living, walking example of 'don't let your age define you'. I had my first baby at forty, my second baby at forty-five – the day before my forty-fifth birthday – I got my first international book deal at fifty, so I think for me the most surprising thing that happened to me at forty and beyond, was everything I thought wouldn't happen for me ... happened for me.

— *Frances Whiting*

mother felt being forty provided a level of maturity throughout the entire process; I never panicked, didn't put my wants ahead of the baby's needs, and have trusted my gut instincts. Having watched everyone else around me have children and struggle with newborn life, my eyes were wide open as to what to expect, all thanks to being older.'

Her bonny little daughter is eight months old now; a grinning ray of sunshine who is yet to understand she is a dream come true for not only her parents, but for everyone who witnessed the years Andy put on a brave face whenever she spoke about a future without her own child in it. But every so often, when she looks at her oh-so-cute cherub, I can still see a look of wonderment cross her face.

'For a long time, I felt she was on loan – like someone else had given me their baby to look after, but that has dwindled over time,' she explained. 'I am utterly amazed she is here. Yesterday, my husband drove past our obstetrician's office on the way to work and called me from the car just to say, "Can you believe we have her in our life?" Getting up in the middle of the night was so much easier when we felt so lucky in the first place.'

Heidi's story
Sarah

My friend Heidi – whom I actually met through Andy – had all four of her children at the advanced maternal ages of thirty-seven, thirty-eight, forty and forty-two, and each experience was incredibly different. Let's start at the beginning.

Heidi met Ned at thirty-three; quickly realising they were each other's person. After travelling the world for a few years, they decided to put having children ahead of having a wedding. The biological clock was ticking, and there was no time to waste – especially as Heidi's mother and aunt hit menopause at thirty-nine and forty, respectively.

Within three months, then 37-year-old Heidi was up-the-duff. It was an easy pregnancy – although that preceded a traumatic birth involving failed suction attempts and forceps – and her first daughter Amelie was born at forty weeks, a perfect creature with a rollicking cry.

As an only child herself, Heidi knew she wanted more than one child if possible, and a year later, quickly fell pregnant again. This birth was the polar opposite.

At 6.44 p.m. on 7 December 2011, Heidi and Ned's second daughter, Sophie, was stillborn at forty weeks and six days' gestation. It felt incomprehensible. The day earlier, her heart had been beating strongly on the monitor in the obstetrician's rooms. However, as some point in the early stages of labour the following morning, Sophie died due to an accidental placental abruption, which meant it detached from the wall of uterus and stopped her supply of oxygen. She was born four hours after her parents were told there was no longer a heartbeat. Another perfect creature, who looked identical to her big sister, but who would never cry.

They spent twenty-four hours together with Sophie in hospital, cuddling and talking to her before the inevitable time came to leave their baby behind. The grief was overwhelming, coupled with not only having to cope with standard post-birth recovery, but the added physical trauma of being in a body primed to nurture a newborn while feeling completely betrayed and bereft.

'When people found out Sophie was stillborn, it's like they were in disbelief she still had to be physically birthed,' Heidi said. 'Um, hello – you can't just magic the baby out! That was then followed by all the typical elements of a vaginal delivery: a swollen stomach, six weeks of bleeding, painful engorged breasts even while taking tablets to stem my milk supply, plus looking in the mirror every day and seeing the reflection of a woman who should have her baby.

'We held her funeral the following week. It was a closed casket, but at the last moment I wanted to see her again. Just me. Just her. Just a private moment together with no one else present.'

Then came the frustration and anger around why Sophie died. In Heidi's words:

Society is very happy to tell you you're a geriatric mother – and how generally speaking it's simply harder to conceive and there's a higher risk of genetic abnormalities, but we were not told of the massively increased risk of stillbirth.

I wish I had known even about the possibility of this outcome. It was never once hinted to us. And although our only known risk was my age (thirty-eight), I wish we'd been told this statistically meant a one in 2000 chance of stillbirth at thirty-nine weeks, a one in 500 chance of stillbirth at forty weeks, and presumably at forty-one weeks the rate would be significantly higher again.

Instead at thirty-eight weeks, we were merely given a choice by our obstetrician: to induce on my due date (1 December), or one week later. It was up to Ned and me to decide and, naively, we thought there was greater value to wait for the birth to be initiated by the baby. Everyone knows that's the best outcome, right? No risks or adverse outcomes were discussed, so an induction was booked for 8 December at forty-one weeks.

As it turns out, I didn't need to be induced and went into natural labour the day prior. There was nothing alarming about the early stages of labour, other than the fact I had a constant dull period-like tightening of my abdomen, lower back pain, and the more intense pains were not at all regular. I had no bleeding or sharp extreme pains, and no reason to feel concerned.

Once we were at the hospital, the midwives started a routine check and were unable to pick up the foetal heartbeat – the first time we had any idea something may be wrong. A midwife left the room to get the on-call obstetrician who returned with an ultrasound machine. The horrible reality hit us when we could clearly see her heart wasn't beating. The words 'I'm sorry' were all we needed to understand our baby had died.

I don't blame any individual person for the death of my daughter, but we need to provide parents with known facts and evidence – not to fearmonger but to empower them to make informed decisions, such as planning the timing of the birth.

I wish someone had told me that in fact my age did put me at risk and said, 'As a geriatric mother, there is a higher risk of stillbirth, it's safe to deliver from thirty-eight or thirty-nine weeks –'

*It's obviously easy to say in hindsight, but we would absolutely
have chosen to induce on Sophie's due date or earlier.*

She started trying for another child three months after having Sophie,
and married Ned the same year.

'It really annoyed me the way people would say, "Oh, well, you fall
pregnant so easily you can just have another one",' Heidi said. 'Even
though I desperately wanted another, it's difficult to explain that urge;
you can't simply replace a baby with a different one.'

However, despite rapidly conceiving in her two prior pregnancies,
nothing happened for several months. At thirty-nine, Heidi was
referred to a fertility specialist after test results indicated her remaining
egg count was almost at menopausal level. On the fifth and final
month of Clomid – an oral medication that stimulates the ovaries
into pumping out more eggs at ovulation – Heidi fell pregnant –
oddly enough on 1 December, Sophie's actual due date a year prior.

Understandably, this pregnancy was an anxious one and she
visited a grief counsellor throughout. Until there was a breathing
baby in her arms, Heidi couldn't relax. 'I would see carefree pregnant
women and think "I *used* to be like them", but at the same time I'd
want to scream: "DON'T YOU KNOW WHAT CAN HAPPEN?!"'

Then, another challenge. The first trimester blood test, combined
with Heidi's age, revealed a one in 165 risk of Down's syndrome.
Anything less than one in 300 is considered high, and additional
testing was offered. At that point in time, Australia's non-invasive
prenatal test (NIPT) was only available in one state and would have
cost thousands of dollars, plus flights and accommodations. The
option of an amniocentesis, which involves extracting and testing
amniotic fluid from around the baby, carried a miscarriage risk.

Heidi and Ned had already decided they would not terminate
the pregnancy regardless of results, and so declined all further tests.

Having experienced the blow of losing Sophie with no knowledge of stillbirth statistics, the pair felt further confronted around the medical and societal pressure of possibly having a child with Down's syndrome.

In Heidi's words again:

It seems counterintuitive that labelling a mother as high risk for Down's syndrome warrants concern and further tests, while the risk of one in 500 for an outcome that will result in your baby dying never even gets a mention.

Every single mother is made aware that she has a risk profile, and that Down's syndrome is a reality for some babies. Surely, we should be treating stillbirth with the same respect – as even if the risk is extremely low, having the discussion raises awareness with the parents that this horrifying result didn't end in the 1800s and is not reserved for third-world countries.

Although a planned induction was scheduled for thirty-nine weeks, Heidi went into labour at thirty-eight weeks. At the age of forty, and twenty months after Sophie's birth, she delivered their third child, Max. He was perfect.

'I felt immense relief and while it was emotional, it was a completely different experience,' she explained. 'We knew we were having a boy, and I was initially disappointed in a weird way because I always thought of having two little girls, but by the time Max was born, I was 100 per cent accepting of him not being a Sophie-replacement and had let go of having only daughters running around the place. There were times when he was sleeping and I'd just have to hold him and rock him and see him and feel him: my healthy little baby.'

Heidi is open about the fact Max wouldn't have been born if Sophie had lived, and how difficult it was to make the decision to not have any more children. Given her established 'geriatric mother' status and the scientific unlikelihood of conceiving without IVF, she and Ned weren't using contraception when – BOOM! Another baby was on its way. They were over the moon and, at forty-two, Heidi gave birth to their fourth child and third daughter, Zara.

'Then, I finally knew our family was complete,' she said. 'I'd been pregnant for 159 weeks from the ages of thirty-seven to forty-two and was basically throwing maternity and baby clothes and cots at anyone who even mentioned wanting kids!'

As a parent advocate with the Stillbirth Centre of Research Excellence, Heidi is driven to change the narrative around stillbirth and has spoken at medical symposiums, conferences, and even at Parliament House:

> *Despite all the years that have passed, and all the speeches delivered since losing Sophie, the hardest question to answer is still when strangers ask how many children I have. I say four, and if they ask their ages I'll say, 'My oldest is eleven and my youngest is six'. That way, Sophie isn't omitted, but I don't have to explain it further.*
>
> *I still think of her every day and wonder what she would have been like. Would she have blonde hair and blue eyes like her sisters? There are triggers, of course – I still struggle with newborns – but I've learned to compartmentalise my grief and imagine a box in my mind where all the thoughts and emotions for Sophie are placed. Sometimes I open the lid and let the feelings out, but now know when to close the lid.*
>
> *Ned and I remember Sophie every day and, even though she isn't with us, she remains an important and much-loved member of our family – as a daughter, sister, granddaughter, niece and cousin – and always will.*

Now forty-eight, Heidi's matter-of-fact about being an older mother and, although recognising her energy levels may have been different if she'd been a younger parent, she's thankful for how life turned out.

Many of her long-term friends – met during uni years or hospital physio rounds or world travels – now have children with driver's licences and fledgling careers, placing them in the stage of life that still feels like light-years away for Heidi, with three children in primary school.

'My "old" friends are still gold to me and we've been together through thick and thin, but by default I've also made another group of younger friends through the school community and although I don't *feel* older than them – maybe that's my immaturity, ha! – I'm definitely choosier about making new friends these days,' Heidi explained.

'I have a lot more life experience and had the chance to travel the world for eight years before having kids. If I'd had a family younger, I wouldn't have given myself that chance because what I know as a parent is I put the kids' needs and wants as a priority over mine. I've had my youth to be inwardly focused, now my life's about them.'

My mother and me

Sarah

I count my blessings to have a close mother–daughter relationship. Dare I say, sometimes too close, perhaps influenced by my family position as the eldest of three daughters. I've always been an open book and my sisters, Rach and Jen, would often cry, 'WHY DO YOU TELL MUM EVERYTHING?'

....

Sidebar: But twenty-three years later, I stand by my decision to dob on Rach for nicking slips from nuns and forging notes in a bid to wag school: middle kids are mysterious, disobedient creatures to eldest children.

....

For the majority of my life, any decision made had a dollop of 'what will Mum think?' thrown in. Like, multiply standard Catholic guilt by about ten, and *et voilà*. The thought of disappointing her (and Dad, of course) was enough to keep me on the straight and narrow. She's been my conscience since forever, and the original imbue-r of my confidence.

But just to be clear – Mum's not one of those parents who ever automatically thought the sun shone out of her children. No. No. No. That's because she was a teacher, and any offspring of teachers reading this know *exactly* what this means: over many years they've dealt with so many students' parents who believe their spawn to be golden little angels when they were, in fact, the devil incarnate at school. They subsequently treat every child – even their own – with a hint of suspicion. It's incredibly unnerving, and I do not doubt my teenage friends were slightly terrified of her in a healthy way.

Now sixty-six and retired, Mum will still take an instant, unapologetic dislike to adults she believes would have been naughty in class. (Unnervingly, usually right.)

And you know how teachers ask a question, but then do that weird thing with their eyes and head position while waiting for an answer and leave you hanging, but then they answer it themselves? Well, that happened at home, too:

- 'Did you just say *youse*? (eyes widen) I don't see any female sheep around here! *Youse* is not a word, Sarah.'
- 'And where do we put our uniforms? On the (eyes widen) … hangers.'
- 'If you want me to drive you to the party, what do you have to do? (eyes widen) Tidy your room.'

Just because we wanted something, doesn't mean we got it. For example, at the end of Year 11 we moved from regional Queensland – where I'd attended a co-ed college – to Brisbane. It meant my Year 12 was at a flash all-girls' school. (You can always tell a fancy school by how unflattering the uniform colour combo is, can't you?) Anyway, it was a whole different ball game.

A couple of months in, I politely asked Mum to *please-oh-pretty-please* buy me a pair of R.M. Williams boots – just like the city girls wore – as sketching the Stussy 'S' on Dunlops was not *de rigueur* at my new school. Instead, she rocked home with a pair of eucalyptus-scented hiking boots. It was an early lesson in social resilience.

The only other thing to add is wearing those mustard-yellow clodhoppers probably meant a lot of people thought I was involved in an illicit affair with a koala for the duration of 1997.

Although – I'll tell you what I did always get: Mum's unwavering belief in my talents. When it came time to go to university, it was Mum who assured Dad they were doing the right thing letting me study theatre – I'd been offered one of only twenty-five places for a highly regarded Arts degree. Dad – ever the introverted pragmatist – worried about my future and getting a steady job, and he thought it surely more sensible to join the police or become a nurse and have stability, forever and ever amen. But Mum was adamant her daughters should try to create enjoyable careers based on a passion.

Did I end up working in theatre? No.

Do I regret doing that degree? Also no.

Because years later at thirty-six, when ten-plus years of corporate communications life switched into a surprise career in radio and live events after meeting Lise, all those skills came in real handy again. Thanks, Mum.

Reflecting on my formative years, and despite living under the suburban dictatorship of a History/English teacher (which included never being allowed to watch *Home and Away* or buy *Dolly* magazines – a knife to my teen heart), it was a safe, loving, and happy family life.

If we got in trouble, we deserved it.

If we could do better, we were told as much.

If we did well, we were praised.

Our love language was a sense of humour. Teasing, heckling and laughing was constant.

Mum would call the three of us to the bottom of the stairs just to throw dirty laundry on our heads.

She banned us from feeding a stray ginger cat outside – '*Don't you dare give it food, it's a big tomcat and he'll spray everywhere*' – only to eventually end up sharing Vegemite toast in bed with him for the following decade.

Anytime we all went to Mass as a family, Mum would separate us from Dad because we'd be chortling too much, desperately reshuffling us in the pew – a mash of limbs and bums swapping seating order in a one-metre space – while hissing 'Jesus is watching you all' under her breath.

At around forty-six, Mum once stormed upstairs in a fit of rage – what triggered it is a mystery – but it was a frightening sight: her permed bob bounced up and down with every stomp, her lips were sucked-in and thin, she was shaking in fury, the yellow flyswatter was waving in her hand, and at the top of the stairs outside our bedrooms, she started madly smacking … the wall.

Mouths agape, Rach, Jen and I watched as every syllable of 'YOU-BLOOD-DY-KIDS' was punctuated with the slap of the swatter. And we couldn't control ourselves. Mum looked so incredibly ridiculous we began giggling – which made her more annoyed – and little Jen was like, 'Oh my god, what are you doing?!' – until all four of us ended up in fits of hysterical laughter.

....

Sidebar: When I asked my sisters for their strongest memory of Mum, both immediately replied: 'the flyswatter!'

....

Why is that memory so vivid? Because Mum actually lost her cool in that moment? Or because it's a gift to our adult selves to remember her losing control … and it being a happy memory? Or maybe because we saw someone older and wiser managing to laugh at herself, along with everyone else? Perhaps all of the above.

For Mum, it holds a different memory – a tipping point – and one I never realised until penning this piece: 'Sarah, you've made me sound like an absolute loony! The flyswatter incident actually made me realise something was very wrong with me, because I'd never reacted that way with you girls; I was always calm and even-tempered. I went to the GP soon afterwards and found out my thyroid levels were completely off the charts.'

Sidebar: The doctor discovered she had a benign tumour on her thyroid gland, which was removed, along with half her thyroid, plunging her into hypothyroidism almost overnight, and the beginning of years of frustration trying to figure out her new normal.

The other thing to mention about Mum, is she was/is an absolute machine. In my experience, it's a characteristic shared by many Baby Boomers. There's a willingness to roll up sleeves and get a job done, not ask/pay anyone else to do something they can, plus practicality, systems, order ... and a dash of 'In my day, I did *everything*' love/hate martyrdom.

Looking back at everything Mum managed, I feel tired for her. She once said her generation fought for mine to able to do *anything*, but we ended up doing *everything*. I heeded her further advice to not be seen as too capable, as it means people will expect you do ALL. THE. THINGS for ALL. THE. PEOPLE.

I watched Mum do it all ... and it's the one thing I never wanted to emulate. Honestly, I don't even think I could.

The biggest gift we can give to ourselves as women – especially in mid-life when we've got kids, and we've got careers, and we've got elderly parents; we're managing so many things – is to give ourselves time for ourselves. I don't adhere to 'we don't have the time'. What I adhere to is that we haven't carved out the time. We haven't yet decided 'I am important enough to give myself the time to work out what I want to do with my life'.

So many of us have the social overlay that our currency and worth is measured by how available we are. We've grown up with the idea that our worth comes from saying yes to everyone and being available to everyone. And part of our emotional burden

– that emotional load – is trying to make everyone around us comfortable and happy all of the time. Even saying that makes me exhausted. Could you imagine trying to make everyone around you comfortable and happy all the time? I don't see that it's my job to make anybody happy. That is not my role in life.

I think a lot of women are still operating, consciously or unconsciously, on being a good girl, a good woman, a good daughter, a good wife – and I very much subscribe to being good enough. Just good enough, which gives me a lot of freedom.

— Kemi Nekvapil

Life in my forties

Beryl, Sarah's mother

Turning forty meant very little to me. I felt no differently about myself to what I had done in my thirties. Nothing changed. I still looked the same and felt the same mentally. I was always busy, but my energy levels were very high. I took pride in the things I did. It wasn't until I got sick with thyroid disease in my very late forties that the apple cart was upset. So, my first message to all forty-plus-year-old women is always ask for your thyroid levels to be checked regularly, especially if you have a family history of issues.

My main priority was my children – always was, always will be. When I turned forty, my daughters were fourteen, ten and six. My husband was a fly-in/fly-out miner in Papua New Guinea. During my early to mid forties, he came home every six weeks for ten days. We did this roster together for seven years. (Then for another sixteen years, he was away in PNG for sixteen days-on and ten days-off.)

I taught high school part-time from when I was thirty-six to my early fifties. I virtually did everything for myself, by myself. Nobody helped me, but I was well equipped for the task. Actually, I revelled in it. Women of my generation were totally different to the current ones. Mind you, my talented post-war mother had set me a high standard to follow, and I had also been schooled by no-nonsense nuns who demanded obedience and strict routine. As soon as I had my first child, it all just kicked in like clockwork.

In my early forties, I lived in a large regional town where everything was a mere ten-minutes' easy drive. Here, I had a broad spectrum of female friends and colleagues. Maybe a couple of the doctors I knew had weekly cleaners, and they certainly had home nannies for their children, but for the rest, we did not outsource to others for anything. We did our own housework, shopped, cooked home-style meals with little dining out or take-out, entertained in our homes. There was still a 'treat like' feel to going out to dinner, usually reserved for special occasions. We had discovered the coffee shops though, and after-work coffee was a regular outing.

Gardens were still big for everyone during my forties. It was my downtime and relaxation. It is only in recent times that people have reduced their city yards to a postage stamp size and live predominantly indoors. I honestly don't know how anyone can stand it! I *LOVE* having a garden. You need to literally smell the roses! Gardening, mowing, pruning and weeding is also the *BEST* form of exercise, both for mind and body. You can get 'mentally' lost in gardening.

When I was about forty-six, I got an ironing lady. Up until then I still, as I had always done, looked after everything to do with the house and yard, including pool, but I *LIKED* doing it. I found it easy as I am an incredibly tidy and organised person. My mantra has always been: a place for everything and everything in its place. My message number two to women is to follow that mantra and you will have more chance of enjoying your life. Untidiness and disorganisation make life more difficult and rob you of precious time.

By my late forties, I was living in Brisbane, Queensland. Life in a city has a very different pace and my amount of free time was reduced by the travel time. Two of the girls were older and far more demanding, one in particular. I certainly did not control my world in the same blissful way I had done when they were younger.

The busier I saw the working women around me become, the more I saw them struggle to fit everything into their working day. I did not work when my children were little and had ten years as a stay-at-home mother. There were heaps of other mothers at home too. There was playgroup each week, tuckshop, P&F Committee and fundraising. They were great years! My era still had freedom of choice in this matter. Nobody expected us in the workforce with little ones at heel.

Unlike in my forties, your generation have been tightly woven into the economic fabric of society – expected to work double shifts, raising young children while simultaneously being employed outside the home. Some men have stepped up to share the load, but there are many who have not. A man's wage alone will no longer support a family. Women have lost their right to choose home over work. When I chose to stay out of the workplace with small children, we were able to survive on my husband's wage, which, at that time, was just an average scale. Anything I earned after returning to work just allowed us to get ahead more quickly. My husband did not expect me to work. Now it's a given.

By the time I went back to teaching it had become even more demanding than ever. My own kids were delightful when young. However, perhaps being a teacher stood me in good stead for being in touch with growing teenagers. I knew what they could get up to in a peer group mentality. But nothing quite prepared me for dealing with teenage defiance from my own child. I hadn't expected it and I floundered. So, I sought professional wise counsel from others – some things you just can't do on your own.

In saying all that, I count myself blessed that I did not raise my children in the time when access to the internet was readily available via phones. In my forties, we did not have that level of worry to contend with.

One thing that I've noticed *NEVER* changes, no matter what age or generation you are, is the need for fellow female friendships. Women seem to be wired to support other women. It is such a blessing.

Now to another topic, body image and worries in my forties. In short, I can't recall even thinking about it. Nor can I honestly recall talking about it with other women. I know some needed to diet to maintain weight, but gyms, boot camps were foreign to us. Sport was still popular with many. Hair *WAS* important to me. It's the only thing I've ever been prepared to pay someone to do. I've never had a facial, manicure, pedicure or so on. I believe they were considered to be special treats, like a gift voucher present, rather than a regular occurrence for women back then.

And where did my husband fit in to all of this? Blissfully unaware of all that I did because he came home to a well-ordered home and, generally speaking, a happy wife and mother. I would have liked more praise and recognition for the excellent job I did, but that was not in his male nature. He's from an old school era. It actually wasn't until he retired and has watched his daughters' working lives that he perhaps has had a lightbulb moment regarding me and what my life entailed.

Yet another topic you may find interesting is my experience of being a woman in the workplace. In all the years I worked, the only harassment I ever knew came from a female subject coordinator. She was a two-faced, belittling woman who undermined my confidence and position, and did it to others, too. Nastiness and a controlling disposition for power belong to both sexes, I'm afraid. I was always treated with respect, helpfulness, and equality by my male workers in my own experience.

It was only when my health faltered that I faltered, and working/home/city life became a burden for me personally. I did what I believe to be a very wise thing: I took responsibility for my own health and, in my early fifties, I went back to live in the country. Back to a quieter, slower pace of life. I got off the treadmill.

The interview

Lise

A decade ago, in my early thirties, I saved an article that's lived on my computer desktop ever since. At the time, I was steering my weary self through the stupor of early parenthood, incapable of much critical thinking beyond testing the merits of putting the Bonjela tube in the fridge, but something about this piece compelled me to drag it into the folder I'd aptly named, 'When the fog lifts'. To be revisited at a later date.

In my forty-first year, a whole ten years later, that time did come.

The article invited readers to interview someone they love about their life. A series of thirty or so questions aimed to get to the heart of someone's story and who they are in the world.

Perhaps it was the stiff cocktail of interviewing well-known women for our podcast, mixed with the sudden loss of my husband's father, poured over the rocky realisation that there were many things about my mother, now aged sixty-five, that I just didn't know, that made me want to pursue the idea of interviewing her.

I wanted to ask Mum what was important in her life, what she wanted us to do and know after she was gone; what she thought was the secret to a good life; how she was in her forties; how she felt about her marriage in those years, her mothering, her friendships, her career, her passions, and her worries. Life advice from the woman who raised me. Undoubtedly the greatest heirloom I would ever receive. Something that would always connect me to her.

Because how else do you honour someone, if not by showing interest in them?

For so long, since leaving my parents' nest in my late teens, I was self-focused. Normal, I know. To be expected of a young adult, finding her way. Discussions always revolved around my roommates, my adventures overseas, my new love, my future goals, my life, my husband, my kids, my work, my tonsillectomy, my schedule, my week, my life.

I think you hit forty and you realise it's time to shift your gaze from your bellybutton to the women who stand before you, waiting for the day you'll ask them about their life, their experiences, their learnings. This is the real passing on and getting of wisdom.

I've chastised myself for asking complete strangers about their fifth decade before even asking my own mother. I leaned in and absorbed the tales of women I'd never met, who I shared no connection with, while being blind to my own flesh and blood's life experiences. In a weak attempt at a carbon paper metaphor, I'm the yellow sheet and Mum is the white, her life lessons waiting to be transferred via a shiny, carbonised sheet.

I assumed I knew Mum's story. But until you sit down and take the time to ask and listen, not as mother to child, but woman to woman, what you think you know may not be so. If nothing else, this will have brought me closer to my mother. For those of us blessed with a good parent or carer still earthside, perhaps it will encourage you to interview someone you love. It was an immense privilege to have this conversation with my mother. As we chatted there were some quiet tears, many deep belly laughs, even some discomfort at times.

So, this is my love letter to you, Mum. I haven't always had the words, or the sensitivity, to tell you that the way you've lived your life has, and will, continue to inspire me. Wordlessly, your values, grit and kindness are my true north. With each year I mature, I want to spend more time with you, listen more and carry forth your legacy. You are my ultimate teacher.

1 What did you love to do as a kid?

I loved to play with my dolls. Brushing their hair. I loved it so much.

2 What do you remember most about your teenage years?

I remember having my first conflict with Mum, because I wanted to wear clothes she didn't find 'proper', like short shorts, or low-cut tops. I was told I'd look like a floozy. Of course, I said nothing in reply, but it shocked me and stayed with me. Her incorrect judgement of me shocked me. I understand it was likely fear.

3 What were your dreams growing up? What did you aspire to become?

I never had huge ambition. It was an era where girls didn't have as many options and opportunities, compared to today's youth. And living on a small island (New Caledonia), it was even more limited. I just followed the course, and I was content. I had a happy childhood, so I was satisfied and happy just as I was. I didn't aspire to more.

4 How did you choose your career and what was your favourite part about it?

My whole career I worked in the tourism industry. It's what I wanted to do because I like being with people. The thought of being around people during a joyous and exciting time in their lives – travel, holidays – thrilled me.

5   What made you successful at work?

My natural ability and ease around people. My clients liked me. I'm a people-person. I'm a highly organised and efficient person, but above all, it's how I related to people, naturally and with authenticity. Back in the day, people wanting to travel would sit at a desk in front of me and say, 'I have two weeks up my sleeve. What do you suggest? What do you think?' That was a dream for me. Listening and giving advice, learning about them, what type of person they were, what they liked to do – were they outdoorsy, did they like the night life? Communication and problem-solving. The core of my career success was caring deeply about providing happiness for my clients.

6   How does retirement feel?

Every single day, I relish not having to rush. Even now, six years into my retirement, I take a moment to recognise and savour that. It's extraordinary. We are lucky. We have the means to travel, visit new places and change our routine when we need to. If things get stale, we shake it up. We love one another's company. We don't ever get bored of being together.

For us, retirement is about reaping the rewards of the work we put in over the years. The communication we insisted on, with each other, is bearing fruit for us now. Investing in our children when they were young means they made good choices, married good people, are raising their children so that we are all happy and well, and love being together. We appreciate everything, now.

We talk all the time, every day. Every couple will go through hardship. We've all been there. In our case, we fought hard, and it paid off. When you age, you want to see the life you built pay off. You want to live to witness that. A weekend with our grandchildren who are kind and well-mannered and funny and loving – that brings so much joy.

7 What three events most shaped your life?

Meeting your father; your father's mental illness;* having children.

....

Sidebar: My dad has battled with mental illness since I was ten years old – a chemical imbalance triggered by being overworked and overburdened, he wore himself to a shadow. Our family has known some dark times. There were stays in psychiatric care units, debilitating bouts of depression, anxiety attacks on the daily, and years of 'medication roulette' – an exhaustive trial and error of diagnoses and drugs. In the early nineties, mental illness was as taboo as it gets. My dad, the progressive, intelligent, brave fighter he is, spoke up and sought help.

I thank God every day for the gift of his vulnerability. I witnessed the strongest person I know being brought to his knees and fight his way back with professional help, love, patience, and a determination like I've never known. We are the lucky ones, my family and me. But it's important to acknowledge that Dad's fight was largely orchestrated and fuelled by my mother. She fought for him even when he was so far removed from the person we knew him to be. Some seasons, the battles were won. Others saw Mum needing to protect her own sanity – a short separation to recalibrate and re-evaluate – both my parents temporarily felled by a silent, unspoken disease they could never have seen coming.

A bipolar diagnosis finally came (along with the perfect cocktail of medications that he still takes to this day). Mum and Dad clawed their way back to one another, even when they thought their love would surely become a casualty, and I remain in awe of their relationship to this day. I'm so happy and proud to report that my father, now aged seventy-two, has been back to his former glory for two decades. A successful businessman, the kindest of men, community driven, loving, funny, smart – so smart. The absolute rock of our family unit. This story is an important part of my own, and an even bigger part of my mother's life.

8 Were you ever scared to be a parent?

Never. I was twenty-two, so yes, there were moments where I didn't know what I was doing, but I never overthought it. I just got on with it. My mother spent a week with me to show me the ropes, and then that was it. I never questioned myself.

9 What did you do for fun before we were born?

The best times were our years in Sydney, your father and me. We had so much fun. Going to the beach with a big crew, going out at night – we were just so alive and ready for anything, driving old convertible VWs through Sydney, it was such a high. They are my best memories.

10 Why did you decide to have kids?

I didn't even think about making the decision! It was a fact of life. I wanted a family, of course, I wanted children, but I never spent any time considering the alternatives. Of course, we were going to have children! It's what happened after you got married.

11 What three words would you say represented your approach to parenting and why?

Love, discipline, communication. I believe that good parenting requires all three.

12 Is there anything you would change about the way you raised us?

I honestly believe I did reasonably well. I'm happy with the way I raised you both, but sometimes I think I could have spent more time with you. That's my only regret. I don't always love looking at photos of when you were small, because I always think I should have spent more time. I didn't have much patience, maybe? As you get older, you think about that. It's a regret, but at the same time, I know I did my best. We all feel that way, right?

13 How did you take time out for yourself?

I didn't. Not until my forties, when both of you had left home, did that happen. I found it very difficult to disconnect from my responsibilities as a mother, even if you were with your grandparents for a few days. The concept of 'date night' or 'girls' night out' just didn't exist. Occasionally, your grandmother would take you girls so your father and I could get a couple of evenings to ourselves, but more often than not, we would just put you to bed early so that the two of us could be together. It was rarely 'me' time. My focus was on our couple, not on myself.

14 When you think about your children how would you describe them?

Warm, caring, happy, beautiful, wonderful mothers, intelligent women – are all the words that come to mind, for both of my daughters.

15 What message do you have for us that you want us to always keep in mind?

I would tell my children that there are two important things to me – raise your children well but, more importantly, invest in your primary relationship – your couple. Because that's what you're left with, and much earlier than you think. Without that, I don't know, I just can't imagine what my life would be. Keep working on your relationship. Preserve your couple. You'll still be young when your children are likely to leave the nest, and if there's no connection, then what are you left with?

Your children will build their lives and, in order to do that, they will sideline you. And you will feel it, you will. So, without connection and complicity with your partner, what is left?

16 When you think about Dad, how would you describe him?

A rebel. He's always been a bit of a rebel. And at the same time, so gentle, so caring, family oriented, easy-going, easy to live with – even though he can be stubborn.

He is funny, a good communicator – I taught him that. Yes, I did! Because he had no communication skills whatsoever. But now he is wonderful.

17 How did you know Dad was 'The One'?

I just did. I knew very quickly that I wanted to spend the rest of my life with him, even though I was so young. I wasn't even seventeen! Maybe there were others out there that may have been a better match, I don't know, but I've always been happy. I don't know anything else. I had small flirtations as a teen, but I've never had other relationships.

So, I suppose I have nothing to compare with, but I'm so happy with that! For the majority of women of my generation, that's just what it was like. Your father had many women in his youth, but he never lived with anyone, either. We jumped into that phase of life together, for the first time. Your generation has more opportunity to figure out what works for you, what you like, what you want. For us, that wasn't possible.

18 What message do you have for Dad that you want him to always keep in mind?

That I've been happy. That he made me happy.

19 What has made your marriage successful?

Communication and love. Communication was difficult at the beginning. But I always insisted on it. We always got there.

20 Best advice for when things get hard in relationships?

It depends on when it gets hard. For us, it was when you girls were eleven and thirteen. Don't give up. It's worth the fight. It was very difficult for both of us to reconstruct, but we did. Of course, there are marriages where you have to leave – emotional, physical abuse, any of that – but if it's a disconnect, you can repair. That said, there was a time I didn't think we would make it. I did get to that place, I honestly did.

I had left to stay at my friend's house. We separated temporarily – you remember. I was at work one day and it rained, and I thought, 'Oh, I hope he's brought his clothes in from the line'. And I knew in that moment I still cared. I still loved him. It wasn't about the domestic chore, it wasn't that – I just knew my heart would always consider his. I knew it would be hard, but I knew I could get back to where we were.

Men show their love physically, and women, the last thing we want is to go there, to express ourselves that way. That was really hard. I kept telling myself, 'That's the way he knows to show love and connection'. I tried a little bit every day and it did come back.

If you've only been together two or three years, as opposed to fifteen, then that's different, of course. But if you've weathered ten years, I feel you'll be right. A whole decade is a big part of your life. You don't forget ten years easily. Especially if there's been happiness! You don't forget that happiness. That'll get you through. The more time you spend together, the more you secure your future together, I think. Because it all adds up. It counts. There'll always be something you dislike in your partner, something that'll play on your nerves. But the shared moments add up.

21 When you think about our careers, what do you want us to focus on?

I want you to prioritise your family over your careers. Because your family is the most important. You can lose one, and your life will still be happy; but if you lose the other, you lose everything.

22 When you look at our generation, what goes through your mind?

We often say, my friends and I, that you do certain things better than we did. Like time for yourselves to recharge. You know when you need it. We didn't know how to do that. But at the same time, we hear your generation say, 'We have so much on, we're so busy' and it makes us laugh. We think it was more difficult for us. From a household perspective, certainly.

We had a standard imposed on us. We did everything ourselves. Except for being parents today – internet, online, the battles – I don't envy you that. Health was not our priority, not the way it is for your generation – we would smoke; working out never came into it unless it was to lose weight and look good, there were no health and wellness campaigns like there are now. Our attitudes were different. You guys have a better handle on that, too.

23 How would you describe your closest female friendships?

We're so different but our friendship is a two-way street. We know how to give and receive. We know we can count on each other. I know she'll be there. She's the only one I can say that about.

24 How did you look after yourself?

I've always eaten well, we always valued a healthy lifestyle – but that was looking after my family as a whole, though. I always took my makeup off before bed, but I never thought about my personal wellbeing that way, to be honest. Or perhaps that's how I feel in comparison to the women of today. I just didn't think about it at the time. It wouldn't have occurred to me to tell my children not to bother me for two hours because I wanted to read or watch a movie.

Remember that very short Sydney trip you took by yourself to see that musical? Just because you really wanted to, and it brought you pleasure? I never would have had the courage to do that. I use the word courage because I don't see myself as being independent to the level you are. Being alone isn't my thing. I like my own company for a day, but I much prefer being with someone. I like having company.

25 What did you do when you felt overwhelmed or sad?

I always did the same thing. I always told myself, 'There's someone worse off than you. What you're going through is nothing compared to what some are going through.' And that was enough to recalibrate and put me on the right path. I remind myself of my blessings. And it works.

26 What do you enjoy about getting older?

Seeing my children and their families happy.

27 What do you wish you'd done more of in your younger years?

More time for myself, I think. Although, I'm fine with it. I don't have regrets. I never look behind me. There's not much I'd change, honestly. Actually, I regret not studying. Not having that tertiary education. I was one of these teenagers who probably needed a push, and I feel I wasn't pushed enough. I do regret that. I think I could have done something interesting, something good.

28 Fill in the blank: Life's too short ......

... for self-pity. Take action. Make a change. It can be done. I've always thought that action is the answer, the cure, the antidote. Do things, keep doing things, don't think, keep moving forward. It's always been my mantra, my go-to.

29 What do you delight in?

I take pleasure in a glass of wine, talking, reminiscing – they are happy moments in my day. And we take time to sit down, to call a friend or two, every day. And then we'll sit and chat about the conversation we've just had, your father and me, and remember. And I delight in family, of course. Always.

30 What is your guilty pleasure?

Once a month, I'll sit down and watch *The Bold and the Beautiful*. It's so stupid, but I love it. A cigarette with your father here and there. I suppose I should feel guilty. I don't like it ... but I do. I tell myself, I have so few vices, if any.

31 Describe your perfect day.

Going for my morning walk, then coming home to get ready for a nice lunch with you girls or a friend. I love that.

32 What have you learned about other people in life?

That people can deceive and disappoint you. You can count your true friends on one hand, truly.

33 What do you think the world needs more of right now?

Civility and respect. The world of today can be so accepting and tolerant of some things, but then lacks basic respect in so many other areas. Even aircraft travel. Once upon a time people used to dress nicely on a plane, now people are wearing shorts and thongs. Don't forget about the basics. We need more balance. We've lost the balance.

34 What do you think happens after we die?

Because I'm religious, I think we meet the ones we've loved, in some sort of way.

35 What are you most proud of?

My family.

36 What do you find most beautiful about life?

I'm exhausted, Lise! How many more questions are there? You know me, I'm too grounded for questions like this.

37 Is there anything you'd still like to do?

I would like to dance. I always thought I was a ballerina whose career was never given a chance to take off! I just love to watch classical dance, to see that movement. I would have loved to dance. I don't think I'd derive pleasure in doing it now, though. Old people don't look good in tutus!

38 What message would you like to share with your family?

I realise the good fortune I've had in my life – to have had a happy childhood – I've had such a charmed life, really. I thank the heavens every day. I hope that's what you've felt, also, and what your children will feel. It's the goal in life, to be happy. I always circle back to happiness. I've always known how to simplify my life. I'm not that spiritual, that woo-woo. For me, things are straightforward, simple. I don't like complication. I cannot stand complication. It goes against my way of being, of operating. I like things to be simple, to be happy.

For the love of an aunt

Sarah

As a general rule, aunts are fabulous creatures but, dare I say, there's a category of aunts perhaps even more extraordinary: those who do not have children of their own, regardless of the reason. My sisters and I were fortunate beneficiaries of such intense love, and it would be remiss not to mention the completely blinkered and biased love that shone our way from Aunty Kay.

When I was born, Dad's eldest sister Kay was forty-two.

Sidebar: I can only figure out her age because - quick math - Dad became a father at thirty, and Kay firmly belonged to the generation when it was particularly rude to snoop around a lady's age.

It was only natural she would completely dote on the offspring of her youngest brother, who she basically helped raise. It's worth noting Kay had other nieces and nephews, too, but they all lived in different towns and cities, meaning we hit the aunt jackpot.

She'd married in her twenties, but never had children – apparently physically unable to due to a ruptured appendix and subsequent peritonitis when she was young. Back then, women just had to accept their fate, I suppose. Quite the taboo topic being childless (or perhaps child*free*) during the 1950s or sixties, with no investigative testing or array of fertility treatments on the table either. By her early fifties,

109

the man she loved for more than twenty years suddenly left her for another woman.

As kids, we were shielded from grown-up issues, but as adults we learned Kay was so deeply hurt, she refused to ever remove his surname – always being the first Mrs H – and was never remotely interested in finding another love. Perhaps this was another contributing factor as to how much she adored Rach, Jen and me – she had children to love without the responsibility of motherhood, which we suspect suited her just fine.

So many childhood memories involve Kay. Going to the local zoo to stare at the resident monster saltwater crocodile at least six times a year. Sleepovers in her waterbed, where she'd throw the blanket over our eyes during kissing scenes on her tiny black-and-white telly. Her comforting scent of Maroussia perfume combined with cigarette smoke. Her one and only signature dish – a curry that somehow included a banana.

I can still see every corner of her house in my mind, remembering it like it was yesterday instead of thirty years ago. The green colour of the kitchen cupboards. The gold wallpaper in the lounge, and the curtain of clacking beads to walk through from the kitchen to the laundry to the games room to the record player past the pool table. A dresser full of old ball gowns and wigs – petite and perfect for nieces' gentle dress-ups. The stack of weekly magazines to pore over: *Woman's Day, New Idea, That's Life!* Her menacing fat cat and weird little terrier: pets only she adored. Visiting her mother (my Nano) in the nursing home. Chats about who loved Elvis more while we'd watch his movies on a Saturday afternoon, and then play his records afterwards. Buying my very first CD with her – a Harry Connick Jnr collection– in Target, which she'd always pronounce as 'Tar-jay'.

She was calm, never roused, laughed at our jokes, and had all the patience in the world.

She died in 2008, three weeks after being diagnosed with cancer. Doctors never discovered where the primary source started – she had smoked for decades prior to (finally) quitting, plus had the sun-damaged skin so common to her era. Maybe lung cancer. Maybe melanoma. We'll never know.

By this time, I was twenty-eight and sharing a townhouse with my sisters, living a four hour-drive away from the small regional town of our youth, but where Kay had lived her entire adult life. All our grandparents had died – one before I was born, two more by the time I was twelve, and then Nano when I was sixteen. At seventy, Kay was our 'old' person, the one close extended relative who'd known us well from newborns into adulthood.

Knowing she was dying was heartbreaking. I remember sitting outside on the back deck talking to her on the phone. Her voice was croaky from illness. I was desperately trying to hold in my grief, and finally failed. It came out in a staccato of sobs and gulps: 'I *can't believe* this is happening to you – I don't *want* it to – it's so unfair – I *love you so much!*' Her own voice cracked, and there was a pause before she replied with an intensity and tone I'd never heard from her before: 'And I love *you* so much'. We both cried. We both knew.

Kay managed to hold on until we got to the hospital to say our goodbyes. She was so frail, so tiny, and watched us in such an odd way – studying our faces as if to take the memory of them to wherever she was next going. It's truly surreal to hug someone knowing you'll never see them again. Knowing they'll soon cease to exist. That letting go bit? Excruciating. Just before we exited her room, I remember racing back just to have one very last hug.

Three days later, the phone rang, slightly too late at night to be anything other than bad news. It was Mum; Kay had died. Despite our collective sadness, there was immense relief she was no longer suffering.

The moment I took the call, Rach said she could smell the scent of Kay's hand cream in her bedroom. Two weeks afterwards, as I stared up into the night sky while waiting for my husband Wills to drive a tractor over from a farm, I quietly asked Kay to give me a sign she was okay. Seconds later, I saw my first shooting star – it trailed so brightly across the midnight sky and left me with such a sense of comfort and peace. For months afterwards, Jen believed she would smell Kay's perfume around her while she worked in an empty bookstore.

I've lost count of the number of times I've 'tested' her with Elvis – guaranteed she'll send me a song or mention of him within a few minutes. Once, as my own little family drove into Bundaberg – the first time I'd returned in twelve years since Kay's funeral – an Elvis song started playing from the unconnected iPad. We'd been in the car for seven hours and not a sound had come from it.

Remembering Kay still brings me to tears. How much I wish she was still alive to meet my girls and Rach's son. Gosh, she would love them all to bits, too. I like to think she already has met them, in a way. Once, when I visited 'white witch' Beck for the first time (you'll read about her later) with my toddler in tow, she greeted me with 'Thank goodness you're finally here! There is a female presence who will not leave me alone all morning and has been desperate for you to arrive!'

As we sat together at a table, my normally rambunctious, climbing, walking, hectic eighteen-month-old sat quietly beside us in her own little world. Bemused, I told Beck how odd that was, to which she replied, 'Your aunty is playing with her – she loves her and they're totally happy together'.

I didn't doubt it for a second.

The change

Sarah and Lise

As soon as forty hit, suddenly the word *perimenopause* entered our vernacular. Honestly, we had only ever heard about menopause and had no clue its little ugly stepsister might prance into the room years before the clock struck midnight to deliver a zero egg-count. Although you're not officially through menopause until you haven't had a period for twelve months, it may take quite the years to get to that point … hence the *peri*, which means 'around' or 'about'.

With Lise's sister having an early menopause at thirty-nine, she's been on high alert for initial symptoms. We asked our circle of friends how they joined the dots to being peri, given the symptoms, severity, duration, and starting age are all so individual.

Some had little to no indications (periods just got lighter before stopping altogether), but others describe it as a physical and emotional freight train. Here's what a cross section of our ladies offered – bearing in mind some experienced one or two of the below symptoms on-and-off for a couple of years, while others got a super-sized combo deal over a decade or more:

- major period changes, from becoming irregular after thirty-five years of a clockwork cycle, to incredibly heavy bleeding, sometimes leading to iron deficiency
- sweating at night

- insomnia
- brain fog, and generally feeling slow and sluggish
- weight gain
- constant stomach bloat
- an emotional rollercoaster, and mood swings (feeling teary or angry for no reason)
- sore breasts (like, pregnancy-level sore)
- feeling hot all the time, including hot flushes
- itchy and/dry skin, brittle nails
- aches and joint pain
- anxiety and 'not feeling like myself'
- depression
- migraines
- reduced libido and vaginal dryness.

WHOA! This is quite the initial list, and none of this peri/menopausal business sounds like a leisurely stroll through a park at all.

I'm changing things for my PT because I'm perimenopausal. Sometimes when the trainer shows up, I'll say, 'That's not going to happen today. Today you and I are going to walk for half an hour and I'll be on the exercise bike for half an hour, then I'm going to drink a cup of tea and you're going to piss off. That's how it's going to go because I'm bleeding today.'

— Urzila Carlson

Pep's story

On a beautiful autumn afternoon in the Botanic Gardens, a bystander from afar would have witnessed three women talking animatedly under the shade of giant Moreton Bay fig trees; a visual feast that

I'm in a bit of a Battle Royale right now with it all. I've been so focused on raising my kids, having this teaching career with kids, not only was I not focused on what I looked like, I wasn't focused on my health and my fitness either. And that's a mistake I made when perimenopause came calling and I felt like my body started to break down very, very quickly. I put on a lot more weight, my joints started to ache, there was cellulite from hip to knee, you know, the nanna flaps on the arms arrived. And it just seemed to happen so fast. And I've been so used to not having to work hard for any of that kind of physical look, and then, all of a sudden, I was looking in the mirror going, wow, okay, this is interesting! So, it's been a challenge to right that shift for me to be able to look at myself and go, okay, you don't look the way you did when you were twenty-one. You don't look the way you did when you were thirty-five. You're fifty. Is there something I want to change? And if I can't change it, can I find it in me to be okay with this and to love the way I look now?

— *Alison Brahe-Daddo*

swung from heads thrown back with laughter to wiping away tears to gestures so exaggerated it looked like a game of charades between middle-aged ladies ...

We were on a break while emceeing a charity fun run when we'd bumped into one of the event volunteers, Pep. She is a larger-than-life character we'd met a handful of times before who always made us laugh – and this time was no exception. Within minutes, the conversation landed on Pep's white pants and joking about her bravery in wearing said colour to a park, before it quickly pivoted to

Pep spilling the secrets of her menopausal uterus, and it's simply too good not to share.

Pep: Look, I was just tripping along as a normal, middle-aged woman and all of a sudden things started to go a little bit skew-whiff, which I think I put perfectly when I described it to you girls. What was the term I used?

Lise: I think we were laughing too much – I can't remember. It was like 'The Menopausal Flood' or something ...

Pep: Oh, yeah. The word flood was definitely in there, and jaws hit the floor!

Anyway, I was continuing along in life having normal-ish menstrual cycles, and then all of sudden they stopped coming as regularly. I got lulled into this wonderful sense of security that those days had come to an end, and because I honestly believed I was no longer experiencing periods, I wasn't carrying anything in my handbag.

Then, one day, I was at an outdoor concert at a winery – with day drinking and dancing in my white pants – just fantasising about my former life and not recognising I was heading towards fifty, then all of a sudden I stood up and the woman behind me said, 'Hun?' I turned around and said, 'What's up?' and she replied, 'It's about the back of your pants'.

Turns out my floodgates opened. and we are talking, like, when your *waters-broke-during-*

pregnancy-gush level of blood. Just the most extraordinary experience! And of course, it's blood in a public place and you have no means whatsoever to actually control it. I had a denim jacket with me and immediately wrapped it around my waist, but then was faced with cues at the portaloos!

Lise: So, the only thing to do was head home?

Pep: Well, in the middle of nowhere at a music festival, unfortunately there is no heading home, so you've just gotta sort of make do. But yes, you are dealing with something never seen before. It makes that post-birth scenario look like easy streets compared to what I was trying to manage. It was unbelievable.

Sarah: This is really important to talk about because after chatting to you, I then spoke to Mum about her menopause experience and asked if she'd experienced something similar – she said she would occasionally get a heavier period, but nothing to the degree you've just outlined. However, I've heard similar tales from other ladies to know this is very much 'a thing'.

Pep: Absolutely.

Sarah: I'm aware a woman's only technically through menopause after no period for twelve months – and even if you get to eight months clear but then bleed, you have to start the count from day one again – but until you educated us, Pep, I just assumed those periods would be the woman's standard period – but I guess when it's

117

	months and months of uterine lining that's been built up and not shed, I mean, it's pretty clotty, right?
Pep:	(laughs) Look, I honestly don't know how this conversation came up under the fig tree in the Botanic Garden, really because I hadn't seen you girls for a couple of years, so I'm not sure how that was my greeting to you!
Lise:	We loved it!
Sarah:	And I think you started crying because you've got five kids and three of them had all left home in the space of three weeks and you were emotional. Plus, we were telling you how we'd spoken with other women whom that had happened to in the *FORTY* podcast – and you just started tearing up and blaming it on menopause, then the story came out!
Lise:	So, Pep, there was an emotional floodgate that opened, and then the tale of a uterine one …
Pep:	I think I may have had snot – there was nothing dignified about seeing you both for the first time in a couple of years!
Sarah:	No! I love how you said it shouldn't be secret women's business and a shock if it happens. This is 'forewarned is forearmed'.
Lise:	And tell us, Pep – were you terrified? If no one had told you about this [the heavy flow], were you frightened?
Pep:	No, I wasn't frightened. But I'll tell you the weirdest thing that's happened to me this week that I haven't had in a couple of years – ovulating

pains in my uterus. So have I suddenly become momentarily fertile again?! (laughs) I don't know what's going on. HRT [hormone replacement therapy] may help with this sort of thing but I had a mum who had breast cancer twice, so it's been my choice not to go down that path.

There are also hot flushes to get through, which are incredibly intense – I've had to get up *in the middle* of a dinner party and jump under a cold shower, or you wake up in the morning looking like you've just jumped out of the pool after doing laps – and then there's the gushing blood that I cannot describe.

We do actually have to talk about it because for some people that sort of thing *is* going to be very, very frightening when it happens. Well, ladies, apparently it's just part of the process of 'this is yet another thing we have to go through'.

Sarah: We really are ruled by hormones, aren't we? When a girlfriend of mine was going through menopause and having hot flushes, her GP likened it to a car engine trying to start, but the battery's dead. So, you're revving the car and the car's overheating – and that is essentially what your body is doing trying to release an egg. So, your body's going. 'COME ON! GET IT OUT! LET'S ROLL!' and then you end up completely overheating. It stayed with me because I thought that sounds pretty right from what people have described hot flushes as.

Lise: That makes a lot of sense.

Pep: I'm kind of hoping I'm coming out the other end, but it has involved a marriage breakdown and children leaving home. Was that because I've been crazy, or was that just going to happen anyway? (laughs) I don't know.

Sarah: Not to get too personal, but do you think your relationship changed when you were going through menopause?

Lise: Yes, who was telling us about that … it was Kathy Lette. Her marriage fell by the wayside during her menopause and she's come out the other side as happy as Larry with a much younger man!

Sarah: She was saying women's hormones have a massive change that makes them more fiery and feisty, and perhaps means they don't want to put up with the same ol', same ol'.

Pep: Yeah, maybe. Look, I don't know, um – I think I've been really normal but three of the kids have left home, guys, sooo … (laughs) the only ones remaining have to stay because they're minors and have no choice, and maybe you need to talk to them!

Lise: Pep, did you have insomnia? Because for my Mum's menopause journey the most tricky thing was insomnia. She didn't really seem to suffer too much in the other departments, but the sleep has been really troubling. Have you had that?

Pep: Yes, I have had some insomnia, which is weird because I've always been a really deep sleeper.

But – funny story, girls – when I watched
Gone with the Wind as a young woman and
Scarlett O'Hara went to bed that night after
everything had gone to shit and said, 'I'll think
about it tomorrow', I say that to myself when
I'm in the middle of these sort of insomniac
episodes.

Either that, or I get up. I've been known to
do loads of washing, ironing, empty dishwashers,
prepare school lunches, all of that in the
middle of the night. Insomnia is a real thing
for menopause and I've heard that from lots of
women, too.

Sarah: It's so important to ask the older women in your
life what they went through.

Lise: And it's not fearmongering, it's just that
knowledge is power. These things may happen to
you and I, Sarah, or may not: some women sail
through, while others take years and years.
I would rather hear all the stories so then I can
do my darndest to manage it at the first sign and
see someone about it rather than suffering.

Pep: But weirdly, Lise and Sarah, it creeps up on you.
I was about forty-six when I started going through
menopause, which is really early. I'm fifty-
one now and it did creep up on me. You don't
initially really realise what's going on.

What is very important is to go to your GP,
talk to them, and keep having your bloods done.
'Cause they can measure your hormone levels
and know if you do need that assistance through

hormone replacement therapy, or whatever that may be.

It's really important to impart that advice: have a good relationship with your GP. Find one you feel really comfortable with and don't be frightened or uncomfortable about speaking about anything that's happening to you because we do need to know what is going on because there are really significant changes. It's like, I guess puberty all over again – but in the reverse!

Lise: That's really, really wonderful advice, Pep.

Sarah: I'm so pleased we ran into you under the figs and had a cry – and now we can pick right back up where we left off!

Pep: I'm so thrilled to share this!

Lise: Our relationship with you will never be the same – it's better, it's gone to the next level.

Pep: It has; it's really intimate now for you – and everyone else as well! (all laugh)

Sarah: Well, it's a very generous thing to share your own personal adventure with menopause, and we thank you for it.

Lise: I just love women who are so open like this, you know, that's just when you find your people because I don't have time for secrecy.

Pep: We girls have got to stick together, right?

Lise and Sarah: Absolutely!

◉ ◉ ◉

I went to the physio today with tennis elbow ... and I haven't been playing tennis. Far out. I've got plantar fasciitis, tennis elbow, and the physio said, 'I'd like to get you in for a women's health check' – to check I don't have a prolapsed vag. Okay? So that's where I'm at; things are falling apart. She said when you turn forty, tendons don't recover like they used to – and you know how your boobs used to be up here and now they're down there? Everything's doing that. So that's where I'm at.

— *Beth Macdonald*

Katrina's story
Sarah

Katrina is forty-nine and likens her menopause as being 'muddled into a complete shit-show', further compounded with having a twelve-year-old daughter approaching her own tween hormonal dump.

In theory, Katrina feels the fact her girl is also being hit with an onslaught of oestrogen surges should make her more empathetic, but the reality is they 'are both walking emotional time bombs under the same roof'. Despite being able to sit together and rationally explain what's happening in their bodies while parked at opposite ends of Fertility Avenue, Kat also feels it makes for an added layer of mother guilt when her own hormone surges take over.

'I'm the adult. I know and can feel what's happening to me and my rational brain is like, "Stop! Be cool! Calm down! Be a good role model", but these completely irrational reactions just surge through me, and are almost uncontrollable – tears, rage, yelling,' she said.

Her physical symptoms began to pummel her around forty-seven years of age, with hot flushes and extreme irritability being the major indicators. She made an appointment with her GP, who asked if she was experiencing heightened irritability in addition to the other symptoms. Katrina joked she'd been peeved since having kids but knew this went far beyond typical parental fatigue.

'I'm not a crier – and never, ever at work – but once during a Zoom conference with senior colleagues I burst into tears because my computer connection was slow,' Katrina recalls. 'I'd been quietly asking for better technology to do my job more efficiently for months, but never made a fuss to my bosses and just pushed through. It was only when one of the young IT guys said, "I can't believe you've put up with this for so long!" that it unleashed a flood of frustration.'

Her husband of fifteen years, Josh, did his best to understand.

'One night, I heard him downstairs watching *Insight* on SBS, and the panel discussion was about menopause. I joined him on the couch, pleased he was listening intently,' Katrina said. 'I was feeling so chuffed as the key takeaways from the program for me were the importance of having a partner who is supportive and there for the highs and lows. Various women were sharing their experiences, and one casually mentioned how quitting alcohol and caffeine helped her moods.

'At the end of the show, and after all the expert women's deep and honest revelations, all Josh matter-of-factly said was, "Well, better stop wine and coffees, then".'

Katrina saw red and let rip: 'That's the one and only thing you took away from that show?! I have sacrificed my BODY, I have sacrificed my BREASTS, I have sacrificed my SLEEP, I have sacrificed my CAREER for this family for years and now you want me to quit my ONE morning coffee and my ONE occasional red wine at dinner?! You've got to be kidding – with everything I'm going through ...'

And on it went.

HRT got really bad press about twenty years ago when two large studies published in well-respected journals showed an apparent link between taking HRT and breast cancer, and also with heart disease and strokes. And it was used to change the medical management of menopause really, so where women were taken off HRT, women weren't started on HRT, it was used for as short a time as possible and as lower doses as possible following all of that.

But since then, we've gone back over that data and realised it was massively flawed. They used the wrong patient groups – they used much older women, high doses of oestrogen, synthetic oestrogens, women who had been post-menopausal for a long time. And you can't apply that data to the way that we would use HRT currently. So, we now use – and we should be using – body identical hormones that have a lower risk. We use a lower dose, we start earlier, and it's thought now to be much, much safer and also to have health advantages. HRT is very safe.

— Dr Naomi Potter

'He looked like a deer in the headlights,' Katrina said. 'But I'll tell you what – he never suggested that again.'

Kathy Lette's story

Lise:	You seem to be experiencing your middle years with a lot of zest for life, with a lot of passion and love for these years. Is there truth to that?
Kathy:	I think for women, life is in two acts and the interval is the menopause – which is pretty gruesome. But once you get through the menopause where you sweat so much it's like the Gestapo trying to get a confession out of you, on the other side of that is liberation. No periods! No pregnancy scares! Your oestrogen goes down and the testosterone comes up and you get a little bit more bolshy, a little bit more selfish, a little bit more like a bloke basically.

And you put yourself first for the first time in your life as a female, and it's just the most brilliant fun. You don't care what people think about you anymore. Cause you know how women are brought up to be sort of decorative and demure. I mean, I'm sure you girls know what I mean – research shows that if a man and woman start talking at the same time, the woman always pulls back. I mean, we're far too polite. But post-menopause, this fantastic alchemy fuses in your psyche and your body, where you just no longer give a damn what anybody thinks. It's the best, most blissful time of a woman's life. You've got a lot to look forward to.

Sarah:	Ooh, how exciting!
Kathy:	And HRT is rocket fuel for females. I highly recommend HRT because all it's doing is

replacing the oestrogen and the testosterone
and the progesterone that you lose during
the menopause, and if you think about it, in
evolutionary terms, the menopause is a new
phenomenon. I mean, until fairly recently,
everybody would have been dead by about, oh,
thirty-two – either killed in war or childbirth.

Sarah: Oh gosh, when you think of it like that, yeah –
we were never meant to be alive long enough for
our eggs to shrivel!

Kathy: Exactly! Oestrogen is the female friendly
hormone and it's what keeps you feeling juicy
and sexy and energetic, and you just feel like you
are your old self. When the time comes, I mean,
you can muck around with all of that herbal
junk if you want too. But you know, please, why
not just donate that money to a charity of your
choice and just whack on the HRT patch and get
back in the saddle.

Sarah: But then you've explained what happens to men
hormone-wise too, and how that is so different,
the imbalance in male hormones.

Lise: Until you said it, I didn't actually realise that
happened.

Kathy: Well, one of the reasons that the majority of
divorces are initiated by women – and the peak
two times is when the last kid finishes school
or when the husband retires – is because of
this hormonal imbalance, you know, women's
testosterone goes up, oestrogen goes down a
bit, and we're like: 'I want to take on the world!

I want to climb Mount Everest and go up the Amazon and go tango dancing in Brazil!'

But for men, the opposite happens. Their testosterone goes down and their oestrogen comes up, so they want to sit at home and nest. They want to lie on the couch and watch TV! And the women are like: I HAVE nested! I HAVE buttered four thousand acres of toast, I HAVE cooked hundreds of flocks of lambs and herds of beef! Women are like, let me out of here!

But it is a real problem, so a lot of my girlfriends in their sixties are giving their husbands testosterone, they sneak a little – of their own HRT – a little bit of testosterone onto their bloke's skin when he's not looking to keep his pecker up, literally.

Sarah: Wow! That's sounds consensual. (All laugh.)
            I suppose it's harder to get them to swallow a
            Viagra –

Lise: You could crush it between spoons with a bit of
            honey –

Sarah: Or you know when you have to open the cat's
            mouth and you're trying to push the tablet down
            its throat while grunting 'you WILL swallow this'
            while it's screeching and meowing –

Kathy: Just worming the husband! (All laugh.) But the
            best way to stay young is to embrace your human
            Wonderbras. I would be totally flat without my
            female friends. It's your girlfriends who keep you
            buoyant in life, so never turn down a chance
            to go out with your chums. And what I love

about when women get together, we strip off our emotional undies in about 3.6 seconds and it's a psychological striptease that reveals all. Our humour is much more confessional, cathartic, self-deprecating, incredibly candid. You know, we share *every*thing and men would be horrified if they knew what we talk about when we're together! In a way, confessional laughter with girlfriends allows you to strap a giant shock absorber to your brain. If you can laugh at something, it takes the sting out of it.

And because women don't have to compete about how big our clitorises are, we don't have that innate sense of competition in our psyche when we get together. Don't you find when you're with your girlfriends, how hilariously honest it is? And once you know you're not the only one going through something, it makes it so much more bearable, doesn't it?

You just want to know you're not alone.

If a woman does not want to have HRT, I think that's her decision. As long as it's based on fact and not on what she's heard at the pub, or heard her friends say, or read in some scaremongering article on Instagram. It doesn't postpone the inevitable because HRT is controlled. So, the perimenopause and the reason why you take HRT is it smooths out hormones and it basically alleviates those big hormonal fluctuations and replaces oestrogen in a controlled way.

If women choose to explore alternatives and if those alternatives work for them and they are not harmful in any way, then I think it's absolutely fine. It's always going to be the way that some women choose to go there. But there are a lot of people out there making a lot of money from vulnerable women who are taken down very expensive investigation routes and give them very expensive supplements and given very restrictive diets. And that's not something that I would promote at all.

— Dr Naomi Potter

Work

You are going to have different challenges come into your life and you are going to have different opportunities, and you have to ultimately let it sit with you and marinate and see what your internal compass says is the right thing to do and then you have to leap. And then sometimes when you leap that's when the most juicy things in your life are going to happen.

— Catriona Rowntree

We quit

Lise

In April 2021, Sarah and I decided to step away from breakfast radio, a job we'd serendipitously found ourselves in after years of dreaming of a media career that would recognise and celebrate our talents. And yet, just four and a half years in, the dream wasn't cutting it for us anymore.

Our unease had started swirling twelve months prior. We'd said yes to an opportunity on breakfast radio in a southern city close to two hours from our homes. Many people will commute that distance daily, but the 5 a.m. start, shift-working husbands and kids in the mix suggested it would be an impossibly idiotic undertaking. Instead, we agreed on the big wigs' suggestion of spending two days and two nights each week away from home, dividing our time between cities.

The novelty of regular hotel stays, uninterrupted Uber Eats and fluffy robes made us temporarily giddy. Then reality kicked in: 4.30 a.m. alarms, three hours on air, post-show meetings followed by station and listener events – and that was just for show number one. By midday we were starting pre-show brainstorms for our second daily show – a national early breakfast slot we were still contracted to do. Two breakfast shows per day, not to mention the mental gymnastics (and anguish) of family logistics in our absence. What were we thinking?

We'll tell you what we were thinking:

This is it!

This is the step before the big call up, the final hurdle before we get the tap on the shoulder for the gig we really want.

If we show them what we can do, how dedicated we are, then it's only up from here.

The kids are older now. It's doable at that end.

We should be so grateful to have not one, but two radio shows!

We need to pay our dues. We'll just dig deep and show them we've got grit.

That grit turned to shit. Real fast.

Our weeks were a hurricane of calendar reminders, WhatsApp threads, school notifications, trips up and down the M1, FaceTime calls, hotel check-ins, half-unpacked suitcases, all set to the soundtrack of a pre-dawn alarm.

Slowly but surely, our energy and zest went down the toilet. A particular lowlight saw Sarah back on the mics, waif-like, after a five-day bout of gastro, while I sat beside her incubating a nasty case of pink eye. We were messes. Something had to give.

Something funny happens when you find yourself at a career junction between long-held dreams and stone-cold reality. You feel yourself growing anxious and restless, asking 'what's next?' even though significant investment has been made to get you to where you are. It's confronting and uncomfortable. We started opening up to our trusted inner circle, not just about work, but also about the toll it was taking on our relationships, our wellbeing, and our creative spark.

> There was just no balance. I would think, 'I don't know what to do, I don't know what I'm going to do.' I feel like I have to burn my whole life down and build it from the ground up ... It felt like I had to put a bomb under everything.
>
> — *Julie Goodwin*

The lightbulb moment eventually came, and it changed everything. We realised, quite simply, that our goalposts had moved, and maybe, just maybe, it was okay for our dreams to be fluid.

Who says you're not allowed to change your mind? It's okay to desperately want something only to realise once you're there that it may not be for you, after all. Your 'dream job' may only be a dream for three years. And then it might become like one of those weird night terrors you get from eating too much cheese late in the evening. It doesn't mean you're ungrateful, nor fickle. Those are all words that are thrown our way, either by ourselves or others, to keep us in a box. Don't want too much! Don't be too big! Don't appear too greedy, too needy, too capricious! Just be happy with your lot. Ignore that voice in your head, that feeling in your gut that there might just be another way of doing things!

What it took was for Sarah and me to get real with ourselves and take the temperature of our current realities. And so, we shoved that metaphorical thermometer under our tongues and into our armpits and assessed where we were at versus where we wanted to be. Sarah and I are not mercurial people who change our minds on a whim, but our lives – heck, everyone's lives – can burn hot one minute only to go cold the next. And that's okay.

Granted, not everyone can do what we did. Many are tethered to jobs regardless of whether they want to hurl their current work

> Mum has a couple of good expressions. Number one is step off the universe – it works all the time. If you are anxious, or stressed about something, if you're sad, or really worrying about a problem, my mum would always say to me, 'All right, you need to step off the universe'. And that's code for give yourself permission – just for a day or a night – to completely remove yourself from this problem. Step off, step away from it.
>
> *— Frances Whiting*

situations into a bin fire or not, but we were in a position to blow things up for ourselves. So, we pulled the grenade pin and did just that.

Kaboom.

As soon as we came out with our plan, oh, how the floodgates opened! Friends, colleagues and school-gate acquaintances all joined in the chorus of 'Oh God, that's me! My job isn't serving me anymore. I'm tired of being on the hamster wheel, too!' Speaking out seemed to give others permission to do the same.

It's funny because once upon a time, younger Lise and younger Sarah may have felt ashamed of quitting. A taboo, drama-fuelled verb seen as a sign of weakness – a stamina deficit reserved for the self-indulgent. Today, it feels honest to have put up our hands and named our exhaustion and our frustrations.

And here's the other thing. Even if it wasn't burnout – because Lord knows there are people suffering through far bigger, more taxing jobs than us – the truth is that we were also simply dissatisfied. And, for a long time, maybe it was easier to hide behind 'burnout' because that feels legit, doesn't it? It feels like a valid reason for someone to quit. Whereas plain old dissatisfaction, well, that stinks of privilege.

I suddenly just went, 'I'm holding on to the dreams and the goals of a girl who was twenty, and I'm not her anymore and I need to recalibrate that.'

— *Justine Cullen*

Truth is, quitting may just be the greatest self-care act of my life, whether burnout brought it on, or dissatisfaction made me do it.

So, if your job is wrapping its tentacles around your life and squeezing until you can hardly breathe, then cut that kraken loose. Or at least befriend it and try to tame it. Take it out to lunch. Get real with your kraken. As Sarah said, while we stood on the precipice of The Big Quit of 2021, 'Nothing changes if nothing changes'.

And as I often say in reply, 'Let's do this, binch.'

And so, we did.

There's no 'I' in team

Sarah

By the time you turn forty, you will realise the phrase 'team-building exercise' is, in fact, an oxymoron. In all likelihood, you too have had to endure the torturing endeavour that is a boss's desperate attempt to bring a group of people (who already work too many hours in too-close proximity) closer together. Usually, the aim of the proposed activity involves making you all look like a bunch of fools, and the bonding element comes from discovering Steve from HR is a casual racist, or quiet Maddie from Accounts is a competitive bulldog during grass sprints in the Botanic Gardens.

There is no point taking employees out of an office for anything other than food and drinks. None. Nada. Zilch. People are better when they're fed and watered, that's a cold, hard fact. So why on earth bosses hit the heady heights of middle management and suddenly snap into 'LET'S BOOK A BUS AND PLAY MINI-GOLF TOGETHER' mode is a continued mystery. And sure, when you're young and fresh and still able to enthusiastically nod whenever someone says, 'There's no I in team, right?', you'll play along because hell, it's paid time away from the desk.

Then, post-forty, you may experience the jolt of realisation that team-building activities are like playing in the pits of Hell, use as many avoidance tactics as humanly possible, or flat-out refuse to participate. You have our permission.

Let's take a trip down memory lane to the straw that broke my and Lise's team-building back:

Year: 2019

Age: thirty-nine

Job: Radio

First, you need to know how intense breakfast radio is, and from 5 a.m. to 11 a.m. weekdays, the on-air crew and off-air team are ~~trapped~~ seated in a tiny studio or airlock listening to each other talk about themselves and opinions. This results in intense friendships and relationships very quickly. You know the ins-and-outs of your colleagues lives almost as well as they do.

You would think that's enough bonding time, right?

Apparently not.

Second, it's helpful to understand my position on improvisation around hypothetical situations, which was first formed in 1992 during primary school drama and teachers screeching 'SPACE JUMP'. It's a monumental waste of brain power and energy. And I'm terrible at it.

The mere thought of having to pretend in ridiculous scenarios filled me with dread. (And that's saying something because once upon a time, I had to dribble on myself during a Kabuki performance at uni.) To further prove this point, at nineteen I auditioned to be a children's TV show host and when the director handed me a ball and asked me to, a) pretend it was something completely different and, b) explain the story behind it, I floundered and said it was a teddy bear a little Jewish girl travelled with through Nazi Germany after she was removed from her parents. Excellent vibe for four- to eight-year-olds. The shocked look on his face has stayed with me. I didn't get the job.

I told you the above to set the scene (pun intended) for the day a two-part, team-building day was sprung on us, but without the activity being revealed. The one thing worse than a two-part team-building day, is a SURPRISE two-part, team-building day. Kill me now.

We were picked up from the studio by the promo team in the radio station cars and driven to the first stop. A community theatre. Oh, Christ – no! Anything but this!

We walked inside, where a theatre sports instructor was waiting for us. My whole body started alternating between fight, flight and freeze modes, which manifested as a facial expression not dissimilar to the one time I had to scrape my dead cat off the road: HORROR. Lise – knowing me too well – started overcompensating with enthusiasm (albeit false) as I began to emotionally and physically shut down, which is possibly my favourite friendship characteristic of hers. She's like one of those nesting birds at the beach that will fake-limp to draw predators away from defenceless offspring. Outstanding.

But theatre sports take no victims, and for two hours I had to endure its stupidity, and the team had to endure my lack of poker-face.

What's the point of hitting forty if you *still* have to put on a poker face and pretend to like something you actually hate? I would rather have salted hot chips placed on my retinas than ever have a three-minute conversation test of back-and-forth questions ever again.

Then, once that purgatory was complete, we drove to another Hell pit in the form of an Escape Room. For the uninitiated, these are itty-bitty locked rooms full of obscure riddles that require solving to get the ultimate goal: the escape. Some people love them. These people are also known as freaks.

There is nothing enjoyable about attempting to decode a timesheet to find a number to open a lock to retrieve a key to open a plywood drawer with a poxy calculator and notepad in it. NOTHING.

Again, another ridiculous hypothetical situation, this time with a man named Phil watching us struggle on camera from the front desk … and who can let us out *at any point in time*. Poor Phil did say no one had ever actually pulled a box FROM THE WALL in the hunt for clues, though. (What can I say? My 'enthusiasm' manifested as anger like a Gallagher brother in a hotel room.)

So, while my colleagues madly used their left brain to rationally sift through numbers and complex reasoning, I was the equivalent of a useless blob of Play-Doh who knew *technically* I could get out immediately by simply picking up the walkie-talkie and lying to Phil that I needed my asthma inhaler. Turns out the whole thing was being filmed for social media though so: FOILED.

Honestly, say no to team building. Although the following year, the boss sent all the ladies off for a facial and massage. This experience was very lovely. The only downside was that it too was a SURPRISE, and I was wearing very questionably adhered boob tape and the most grey and misshapen G-string in my entire undies drawer.

Lise, of course, de-robed and was wearing a matching set. Who does that? Who wears matching bra and knickers on a Wednesday unless you are dating someone? I haven't owned a combo like that since 2007! Then, I realised: AHA! She is coming to my rescue – acting like the injured bird at the beach again to give me and my boob tape time to flee, bless her.

That's what friends in your forties are for: in good times, and in bad (team-building) times.

Nice no more

Sarah

NICE [*adjective*]: *polite, pleasing, agreeable, appropriate, fitting.*

For so many years, that was our goal, wasn't it? Being a nice girl. Someone who didn't stir the pot or make trouble; someone who made everyone feel comfortable by not being contentious or contrary. It's quite possibly the ultimate people-pleaser attribute, and a word that needs to be assessed for what it truly means when it comes to describing a person: someone who is easily taken advantage of, and often.

Being brutally honest, we wore 'nice' like a badge of honour in younger years. Oh, the self-sacrifices we made in order to be likeable non-disrupters AT ALL TIMES. Being nice is the social shackles to hide hackles. (Oh, God, that's so good. Make it a meme.)

But, it's true, isn't it? It's always putting others ahead to the detriment of your wants and needs. Nice meant I stayed quiet and smiled instead of speaking up, and shaking things up.

At twenty-three, I signed up to a self-defence program with a group of girlfriends as a fun activity together – with the added bonus of learning new skills. Held on a weeknight at a university, there were a lot of young women in the class, which was led by a grey-bearded man, roughly in his fifties. (I can't recall his name but, for

141

As a black woman born in England in the 1970s, always navigating white spaces, I had to be a good, good, good girl. A good black girl. Because the story I was told was all the people who looked like me (by all the white people around), was that black people were bad. So, I decided I was going to be a GOOD black person. It was internalised racism which I didn't get to unpick until my early twenties. And then over time, probably from twenty to thirty, I spent a lot of time being nice. I spent a lot of energy making sure that no one around me felt threatened if I had an opinion about things. I didn't want to agitate or rock the boat in any way, and I just kind of wasn't living. I mean I was living and having adventures, but I was hiding parts of myself to be acceptable to others so I wouldn't have the experience of being cast out.

— *Kemi Nekvapil*

the purpose of this tale, let's call him Dick.) Over the course, we learned a manoeuvre to defend ourselves if, say, we were grabbed from behind at an ATM. Dick would wrap his arms around our chest, and our trained reaction was to pull down on his forearms to break the grip, while bending our knees to throw his body weight off our back, then drop him over a shoulder onto the mat.

After going for several weeks, it was my turn during class to practise this move with Dick, while the other students worked in pairs, overseen by a younger male teacher. Facing the back of the room, Dick wrapped his arms across my shoulders, which was not where he had put them before. I'm a tall woman, and I asked him to bring his grip down across my chest to do it properly. He did move his arms down – then nuzzled his head into the left side of my neck,

> I'm not even interested in 'nice' ... because nice sounds like you're being walked over. You can be kind. Kind and nice are different things. Nice is about putting up with a lot of shit, I think, and holding your real self back.
>
> — *Rebecca Sparrow*

squeezed my right breast three times, and said 'ooooh' into my ear with each squeeze.

Time seemed to stop: did the man I paid to teach me self-defence skills to protect me from men just grope me? Yes, he did. Somehow, he let me throw him off. What did I do? Absolutely nothing. I was in total shock. I remember shaking, clamming up, not looking him in the eye. Nobody saw it happen.

I told my friends after the class, and never returned for the final few weeks. The pleasant younger instructor eventually asked why I wasn't showing up, and a friend told him the truth. His reply to her? 'Oh, not again.'

For years I wondered what about me said 'you can grope me and get away with it'. Now? Pretty sure I know why: because I was a nice girl, and nice girls don't make a fuss.

> I don't know if it's a female thing or being raised a certain way, you want to be nice. I was saying the other day, when you're growing up, everyone's like 'make sure you don't eat the cake first, make sure everyone else has the cake first' ... don't make anybody else feel bad.
>
> — *Sally Obermeder*

That has slowly changed over the years. I will call out inappropriate or disrespectful behaviour. I once walked out of a meeting when a man repeatedly interrupted me and continually asked if I thought I was better than him. Better than him? No. Better than that situation? Yes.

Now in my forties, I make the fuss. Trust your instincts. Be prepared to walk away from anything and stand up for *everything* important to your values. Nice no more.

It's so engrained in us to be liked. And I remember years and years ago, I thought, that's not what I want my gravestone to say: 'She was liked. She was nice.'

— Kemi Nekvapil

Overwhelm

Sarah

It all started at my favourite local coffee shop, a tiny slice of no-frills suburbia joy, where the baristas are young and chirpy, the chairs are metal and the tables wobble ever so slightly, and every customer is known by name – from the corporates grabbing a latte before jumping on the bus, through mothers entertaining toddlers after school drop-off, to sweaty, fit types spilling out of the gym next door.

When I wandered in at 8.45 a.m. to order a quick coffee, an acquaintance made a harmless-enough quip about how nice it must be to 'work one hour a day'. (At the time, Lise and I were hosting a national early breakfast radio show, which aired around Australia from 5 to 6 a.m. weekdays). I smiled and nodded, but as the line to order reduced in numbers and I stood in front of the cash register, the rage within had started to bubble. One hour a day, hey?

Then, perhaps it was no surprise, when the lovely man who owned the joint asked me how I was, my mouth superseded my brain and flat-out refused to deliver the standard, 'Good thanks, how about you?' reply. No. Instead, I swamped the poor fellow with a diatribe of tasks to be ticked off in the following hours in a blurry recollection of verbal vomit punctuated with, 'I AM ABSOLUTELY EXHAUSTED!'

And do you know what he said? He said, 'Thank you for telling me this, I feel the same way.'

Well, didn't that click something over in my lil' noggin? Suddenly, my inner voice screamed at me to not bottle it up. So, I walked outside with my coffee and toast and promptly told the lady who ran the gym and her friend (whom I'd met in passing twice before) everything that was making me feel GRRR.

It was an out-of-body experience, where I could see them looking at me like trapped mice while trying to enjoy their morning natter, but my tongue was hinged in the middle and would not stop flapping about anything and everything – from the useless nature of parent information nights (I mean, just email it already) to why the hell do we pay $55 for an incredibly un-sunsafe netball dress given everything we know about skin cancers these days, and oh, by the way, the orders are due at midnight and I missed the try-on day and you absolutely cannot go by your daughters' usual clothing size because the netball world operates at least two sizes larger so fingers crossed you choose bike pants that won't ride up their bums for the entire season. And breathe. And leave.

Next stop: texts to friends. Appropriate responses. A collective shout of 'me too' that temporarily soothed the soul but didn't solve the problem. Perhaps it could all be blamed on planetary misalignment – that awfully pesky Mercury was in retrograde *again* and, bugger me dead, that must be it!

Hours later: still annoyed.

The one line that started the internal ricochet kept rising to the top, like the fatty, blobby cream in unpasteurised milk bottles you need to probe and poke for the actual milk to start flowing: 'How nice it must be to work one hour a day.'

There was only one thing left to do – diarise my day.

2.45–3.15 a.m.	Wake up, get dressed, drive to work
3.30–4 a.m.	Pre-show production meeting
4–5 a.m.	Radio show (airing live, 5 to 6 a.m. in Oz's southern states, and replayed in later time zones)
5–5.30 a.m.	Record radio show podcast and post-show production meeting
5.45–6.30 a.m.	Run squad
6.45–7.30 a.m.	Return home, shower, lunches and school prep
7.30–8 a.m.	FORTY podcast edits and copywriting
8–8.30 a.m.	School drop-off, grab coffee and toast
8.30–10 a.m.	Zoom meetings with production companies
10.15–10.30 a.m.	Drink third coffee and stress-eat hot cross buns
10.30–11 a.m.	Prepare dinner based on scraps in fridge (who knew there were recipes for sweet potato and bacon lasagne?)
11 a.m.–2 p.m.	FORTY guest interview research, emails, pay invoices
2–3 p.m.	Clean pool filter, fold undies pile, quick vacuum
3–3.30 p.m.	School pick-up
3.30–4.15 p.m.	Serve afternoon tea and supervise homework
4.15–6.45 p.m.	Kids' gymnastics classes drop-off, tag team with husband, reply to new emails, serve dinner at 5 p.m. and again at 6.40 p.m.
6.45–7 p.m.	Shower
7–7.30 p.m.	Source content for next morning's show
7.45 p.m.	Bedtime

> I can't tell you how many women I've had conversations with who say wouldn't it be lovely if you could go to hospital – just for a day or two, not long – and be sick enough that you cannot have visitors, but not so sick to be actually sick. So perhaps a bit of an unknown thing for testing. Just to get one or two days in bed with your books, meals delivered, a cup of tea, and no one can come near you.
>
> *— Frances Whiting*

Somewhere in the timetable, these were also achieved: maintained relationships without grunting at people (despite reaching the average person's word count by 10 a.m.), ordered the netball uniforms, sent out tenth birthday party invitations, changed the kitty litter and wormed the cat, renegotiated electricity contract because the provider likes to sting loyal pay-on-time customers with a surge in fees and tariffs, and remembered to use both my B5 hyaluronic acid and B3 retinol night serums 'to reduce the signs of premature ageing'. Also succeeded in *not* telling the person who thought I only worked one hour a day to take a long jump off a short pier.

My experience at the coffee shop was a sign that I had a good old case of The Overwhelms, where at some point in your day, your week, your month, or even your year (clap, clap, clap, clap) you make the terrible/wonderful mistake of pausing and realising the amount of life tasks on your plate are actually unpalatable, indigestible, and will likely cause irritable foul-mood syndrome.

And the point, dear reader? When it gets to this point, make the changes you need. Me? Ended up leaving the 'one-hour a day' job and creating a much more palatable career in daylight hours.

*If you carry the mental load, why should anyone else pick any
of it up? You've got to let the mental load fall over the floor from
time to time – then someone will either pick it up, or they won't.*
— Mia Freedman

One of my best friends reminded me others can only meet known
expectations. Speak up and spit it out. Also, no one likes a martyr.

The scathing email

Lise

I have just fired off a scathing email. I am justifiably angry and, for the first time in my life, I'm expressing it.

I've kept it factual, tempering my emotions in favour of cold, hard truths. I have signed off with a *'Ciao* for now', which we all know to be the typed equivalent of a knee to the gut. It says, 'I'm livid but still chill, because I'm right and you're wrong, so watch me sprinkle some casual–cool Italian into this email cauldron of dissatisfaction.'

I've been metabolising my anger for the past two and a half hours, turning it over every which way, inspecting it closely, observing it as I pace around my office. I've played devil's advocate for the opposition, I've flipped the scripts (and the proverbial bird to my computer screen) all to ensure my anger, is in fact, warranted.

And goddamn, it is. I am calling bull. I do not need to be gracious, nor understanding, nor patient any longer. I've been all those things for weeks, and yet, here I am on a Sunday, consumed by other people's inefficiencies and disregard.

Less than a year ago, I would have crafted a very different email. Heck, I may not have even sent one at all. I would have played the nice, easy-to-work-with woman who doesn't kick up a fuss, possibly typing a few saccharine 'All good, guys! It'll get it sorted!', coupled with unnecessary apologies that were never mine to make.

A popular tweet has been doing the rounds lately. It reads: 'Someone recently told me that "difficult to work with" often really means "difficult to take advantage of"' – I haven't stopped thinking about that for weeks. It has tilted my frame of thinking on its axis.

For a long time, I've been driven by the need to be liked. Some will say 'conditioned', and they'd probably be right. My modus operandi was to be proactive and pleasant, easy to work with, and enthusiastic. In many industries – the creative ones in particular – there's a strong stench of 'there's a thousand people who'd kill to be in your shoes' wafting around, which will almost always flare up your anxiety to stay nice, remain likeable, don't make things difficult for the people around you, just be a good little minion or we'll replace you quicker than you can say 'Centrelink'.

Here's the thing with the being-likeable-and-easy-to-work-with algorithm. It is wildly inaccurate because it is wholly one-sided. It will never, ever reflect the fact that sometimes those around you can be inefficient, disrespectful and unresponsive twits. It throws you down a silo, asking you to overlook the incompetence of others, unfairly demanding you to stay neutral at all costs, to numb your reactions, to silence your dissatisfaction.

And you know who's tired of being shushed? FORTY-YEAR-OLD WOMEN.

So, here's a novel idea. If you're rightfully disappointed or upset about something, you can express it. Bonus points if you can weave your high school motto vibes into your delivery – *Fortiter et Suaviter* – 'Strength and Gentleness'.

And by gentleness, I don't mean 'soft'. At forty-one years of age, I also reject gentle as meaning 'impressionable'. I kicked impressionable to the kerb a few years ago. My horse-crap detector is fully functioning, now more than ever. I back my intuition and gut feelings around people and situations. Now, to tell them.

My email is restrained but still packs a punch. It was sent to elicit action not drama. It is firm but fair. I am proud to sign my name to it, knowing it doesn't throw anyone under the bus nor unfairly place blame. Tomorrow, I can look each recipient in the eye, without fear that my words were too harsh. Because they're not. *Fortiter et Suaviter.* It can be done. And let me tell you, it's bloody satisfying when you do.

Keeping up appearances

If you're not at peace with your body – it's your home!
Everything you do in the world, or everything you
want to do, it comes from this place, so we need to get
that in order.

— Taryn Brumfitt

Mirror, mirror

Lise and Sarah

We have some glorious friendships in our lives. Some of these relationships have survived months, even years, without face-to-face contact. Others are tended to weekly. Like Spokey Dokeys on a bicycle wheel, these wonderful women slide back and forth, always in our orbit, always along for the ride. Our friendships move with the tide and change with the seasons. Active or dormant, we value what these women think, deeply.

And so, we wanted to ask them about their own ageing demons. Did they even have any? How were they feeling about getting older? Were they comforted or confronted when they looked at themselves? What are they embracing and what are they challenged by as they age? Deeply personal questions, we know. They rose to the challenge as we hoped they would, quick to share their innermost thoughts and experiences with us when we asked:

How do you feel when you look in the mirror?
Are you scared of ageing, physically?

I really don't look at myself in the mirror much. I mean, I look every day, but I don't really see myself. I take a cursory glance – eyebrows in place, nostrils clean, no random black hairs growing where they shouldn't be, makeup blended if it's a makeup day

– check, and off we go. Generally, I am seeing the day ahead. The list of things I need to do. Prioritising, rescheduling, yelling out to kids to get ready. So, my changing face doesn't often register, and therefore, doesn't usually bother me.

But every now and then, I'll see me. The reaction varies. It depends on the day, the time, the place I'm at in my life when I catch that glance in the mirror. When I really see myself, often, it's surprise. 'Oh gosh, when did that happen? When did I get wrinkles there, change shape like that, put on so much weight? How long have those sunspots been there?' I get a shock. Not a great, exaggerated shock, but certainly a mild one.

Sometimes I'm kind to myself. I see my maturity, my character, my life experience. My ageing as a beautiful thing. Sometimes I'm extremely unkind. I see my weight and it disappoints me. My soft, squishy body as something to be ashamed of. My features as they age looking more masculine, less feminine. I see myself as a failure. They're tough, those moments. But this doesn't happen often. And it happens less and less as I get older and learn what it truly means to be kind to myself. To silence that inner critic because she's the meanest of mean girls. And it benefits no one. Not me, not my kids, not my husband, to see me hating me.

My husband? What does he think of my ageing? Suffice to say, I have learnt that our upbringing significantly influences our opinion of what is beautiful. And it's very hard to change those ingrained beliefs. My husband learnt, from a beautiful mother and two gorgeous sisters who spent their lives dieting and criticising themselves, that being thin is beautiful. This had a very detrimental impact on our relationship when I gained an extra 30 kilograms after three kids, combined with a love of food and drink. It was a learning curve for both of us. It still is. If anything, it's emphasised to me the importance of being okay with myself and not placing my sense of self-worth in someone else's opinion of me. Even if it's my husband, who I trust with my life and my kids' lives.

It's a lot to take in, all that change (good and not so good) every time I look in a mirror. A cursory glance is much easier. Eyebrows in place, nostrils clean, no random black hairs growing where they shouldn't be, makeup blended if it's a makeup day. Check, and off we go.

— Gia, forty-one, Lawyer

I am forty-two. When I look into the mirror I am often torn between the dichotomy of self-judgement versus appreciation. The many moments of joy I have been blessed with – laughter, friends, achievements, and love – that have contributed to the fine lines around my eyes and mouth. Contrasted with the realisation that ageing is hard. That health will inevitably decline, beauty will fade, and that independence will be lost. Life is funny that way. I also just think I need Botox. To keep up, yes. Botox, I feel, is just like make-up – trying to look your best with what you have.

— Daniela, forty-two, Surgeon

When I look in the mirror and see my face, the word that comes to mind sometimes is 'regret' – regret that I didn't apply enough sunscreen over the years and take care of my skin when I was in my twenties.

— Adriana, forty-three, Human Resources

I don't feel positive about my thickening waistline or the fact my once taut tummy is wrapped in thin, papery skin that doesn't seem to fit – a bit like loose cling wrap. I look at my face and I'm starting to look different now. Before I could only see

I'm troubled by the idea that the desirable look for women is one without facial expressions ... The idea of women erasing our facial expressions in the pursuit of looking younger, that doesn't sit well with me at the moment, but I'm also super vain and I also feel super deflated often when I look in the mirror ... because how I look often doesn't match how I feel, and I hear a lot of women saying that, that they have Botox so that their outsides match their insides.

— *Mia Freedman*

it in photos. Now, I see it daily and I'm a little disappointed. I wish my eyes didn't droop so much, and that I had a glow in my cheeks. The wrinkles in my brow are getting a little less funny and a little more serious, urging me to do something. I'll be honest, I'm not taking this ageing thing easily. I'm honest enough to admit that I've been considered attractive over the years. I know it's all relative, but now I feel I can't quite keep up with my peers.

When I say my age, a lot of people seem surprised, and not in a good way, I'm afraid. I'm only forty-four. Every morning I'm lucky that once I apply a little eyeliner, mascara, and a whack of foundation, I get to see the girl (albeit aged) I once was. I like what I see. Sure, she's curvy and is looking more and more like her mother, but nonetheless she's feminine and pretty. She's not hot. She doesn't get the hot looks anymore that she would get several times a day in the past. She gets those from her husband and the occasional octogenarian at the medical centre where she works.

I'm beyond lucky that my husband embraces the changes in my body. My curves are revered, and he still cannot quite *understand why I wear makeup. My beauty is ageless to him. Every woman should have such support and unconditional love. When I asked him how he finds me just as attractive over the years he answered, 'I love that our bodies are changing together across the years'. So, at this point I must accept my ageing. I look to my grandmother and mother, women who I find incredibly attractive for their age. I've also started looking at my body from a functional perspective. It's done so much for me, and it has given me years of good health. For that I'm so thankful.*

— Farah, forty-four, Project Manager

Some days I look weary. Life weary, work weary, wife weary, mum weary. My sparkle has dulled, and I sometimes don't know who it is looking back at me. Lost in the working of life and what I think it should be like. I'm a people pleaser, and when those around me are happy, I am happy. Sometimes it's to my detriment, as there are times I feel I need people more than they need me.

Growing up, I was never the first person invited to birthday parties or sleepovers. I was a farm kid who wasn't rich enough to be a boarding schoolgirl, but also not a 'townie' – I didn't quite fit in. So, I became that country girl who went to the big city with a good personality and a determination to make something of myself. I am an organiser who takes comfort in routine. I always wanted to be a mother. But where to next, once my boys are grown? I actually don't know.

My greatest achievements are my two sons. Watching them grow brings me the greatest joy. I know when they leave home I will be lost – it's that feeling of being needed that I love, and that is the challenge I need to overcome for myself. My forties represent that time in my life when I no longer have to nourish, nurture, and tend to small children the way I once did. That part of my life is coming to an end, and I'm not sure what lies ahead for me. Honestly, that frightens me – I haven't planned for it. Do I want a career? A career change? To study? To work longer hours? I'm not as naturally driven as my husband, so I don't know what the next ten years looks like for me. So, who looks back at me in the mirror? Some days, I honestly don't know who she is.

— Cindy, forty-five, Administration Officer

When I stop and stare at my reflection, I can see that things are hanging lower, sagging, bulging or wrinklier than ever before, yet I've never been more comfortable with, or accepting of, the woman staring back at me. I'm certainly not proud of all I do or say, particularly as holding my tongue seems harder as I age, but I'm accepting of who I am and what I've become. Cranky, loyal, impatient, honest, generous, serious, bossy, silly, supportive, compassionate, emotional, all wrapped up into one.

Some less desirable than others, but all a reminder of my journey and the complexity of being me. Warts and all.

— Sheri, forty-seven, High School Teacher

If you had asked me a couple of months ago how I feel when I look at my ageing self in the mirror my answer would have been completely different. After battling a couple of health scares earlier this year and after fifteen years of parenting, ten of them solo, I was deeply, deeply fatigued and losing my hope that things would ever change. Just over six weeks ago someone gifted me with a wellness program that has been and continues to be completely transformational.

Finally, I am prioritising myself, working on my health and surrounded by a culture of positivity and level of encouragement I didn't know was possible. I'm reclaiming a hope for my future that is no longer a thread I'm clinging to but a belief that I'm walking out and working into every part of my day.

A few weeks into the program, as I began feeling this shift, I wrote out some affirmations and these are now what I see when I look in the mirror.

I see a woman who is delighted in and loved, who sees beauty and light even in the darkest of moments and who lives luminous in the ordinary.

I see someone who never gives up, who is not afraid of the difficult moments in life or the lives of others and who has the wisdom to know when to sit with someone and when to stir them into action.

I see a gentle, nurturing, encouraging mother and I am able to extend those gifts to myself and all I meet, offering presence, comfort and support.

I see a woman living a life of purpose, growing fit and healthy in body, mind and soul, with the courage and tenacity to live a long and healthy life with an active and alert body and mind.

I see someone who is no longer bound by a fear of failure but is free to dream again, to be creative and adventurous and to surround myself with people and structures that will move my ideas from thought to reality.

Hope and belief are what I see when I look in the mirror in this season of my life. I've lived through life-threatening, mind-messing, soul-destroying moments of darkness and I'm not scared anymore. I'm ready for whatever life brings but will also be intentional about how I move into all that the years ahead hold.

— Christine, forty-three, Home-schooling Mother

I was forty-one when I met my second husband. He was twenty-four. A seventeen-year age gap. It was massive. I felt he had his whole life ahead. He was my personal trainer. I thought he was a great guy but nothing more, mainly because he was in a completely different age bracket. I saw what an amazing person he was with all kinds of people, no matter their age. He had empathy, respect. I was able to get to know him on a friendship basis. I'd never met anyone as remarkable as him. He was the opposite of anyone I'd ever met that was his age. I was so confused – on paper, none of it made sense.

I wanted our friendship to deepen and had heard from mutual friends that he liked me as well. We'd all gone out to dinner to celebrate our bootcamp group's achievements. He said, 'You look really beautiful tonight.' I thought he was being courteous because what 24-year-old finds a 41-year-old woman attractive? What would he ever see in me?

Today, five years into our marriage, he says he finds my drive, my ambition, my commitment to my family the sexiest thing he's ever come across. So, when I look in the mirror, I see someone who's risked everything, and I am so grateful for where I've gotten.

I still have so far to go. I self-criticise in my professional life, all the time. On a personal level, I struggle with that, too. It's something we constantly work on – body image, self-talk, how we see ourselves.

I was walking ahead of him the other day, and he said, 'Hey wait up!', followed by, 'Actually, don't. Let me look at that sexy ass!'

I said, 'Oh my God, stop it, it's huge,' to which he replied, 'Don't do that. You have no idea how perfect you are.' Even when I'm tired and I say I look like shit, he tells me I'm beautiful. When you're over forty and your husband is young and sexy as hell, of course I struggle with being positive with myself. I am forty-eight now and he is thirty-one. We talk about ageing; I've talked about Botox because so many of my clients are getting injectables. He's said, 'I want to look at my wife and see you age so beautifully. Before you met me, your age would never have been an issue for you. There will always be seventeen years difference between us. You don't need to freeze time.'

Friends have said, 'Just get it done. He'll never know!' But this is the truest, most honest I've ever been with someone in my life. He knows everything about how I feel about myself, and so I guess I don't need to lie to him, or get it done without him knowing. If I choose to do it because it's important to me, I will do that, but I just don't feel that pressure. I don't need to make myself look younger. He's so embracing of the way I look. The ageing I can handle. Now, I am super comfortable with the lines on my face, the grey hair coming through. I know there's a level of attractiveness to me just the way I am.

— Justine, forty-eight, Stylist

When I hit my forties, that's when I felt the best because I was at my physical peak. I felt well mentally because that's when I felt most confident. I'd gone through some very difficult times, and I was out the other side.

My forties meant I finally had more time to myself. I'd had my children young, so by the time I reached my forties, my eldest was eighteen years old.

Compared to women in their forties today, I feel I was not as concerned with my ageing looks. Constant exposure to social media means you're aware of wrinkles, lines, breasts. I'm part of that generation that didn't question things as much. We weren't as pushed to do it as you are. We didn't question ourselves. It's only now, at sixty-five, that I'm aware and a bit self-conscious, possibly because I have social media myself now?

I wasn't scared to age physically, not in my forties, on the contrary. Ageing felt far away. I remember buying some lingerie that fit beautifully. I felt good.

Now, twenty-five years on, I don't feel like an older woman, but physically that's what I'm beginning to see. But only now. Certainly not at forty!

Now, women in their forties are pressured to keep up with today's societal standards – we want a 47-year-old woman to look like a 37-year-old woman. It wasn't like that for me. I never felt the race, the competition, the pressure if I saw younger women with pert bottoms, perky breasts, and toned arms. I never told myself, 'If you work harder, you can get back there!' That's behind me. You can't anymore. So, you do your best with what you have.

When I was forty and your [Lise's] sister was eighteen, I remember a man looking in our direction, and I realised he was looking at her, my daughter. Losing the male gaze, losing the male attention is a thing. I just accepted it. I do value the male gaze because it can feel nice, right? But when that's over, such is life. That's just my personality.

Your father has always been the one to bolster my confidence. He did everything it took to preserve how I felt about myself. His opinion matters to me, of course it does. But it's always been so positive. At forty-two, you and your sister had left home, your father and I were empty nesters. So, in a sense, I was able to reconnect with who I was as a woman, who we were as a couple. Any evidence that I was old enough to have two grown children was gone – out of my face. We felt young again!

Before that, I would rarely take the time to look after myself, to buy myself nice things. Suddenly, I was able to invest in myself a little more. I spent money to look and feel sexy again – lingerie, my hair, my makeup, my clothing. I felt a hundred per cent myself. I was well. I felt good.

I feel women of today are too focused on their physical value. They're so self-aware. I worry for them when they age – really age. Maybe that's why I've journeyed successfully through the middle years because my focus was never so much on my looks.

— Nicole, sixty-six, retired Airline Manager (and Lise's mother)

When I look in the mirror, I see an older version of my young self. I see a woman who has her mother's hazel-coloured eyes and her silver hair. I see personality lines, crow's feet, and sun damage, mainly from growing up in the tropics. I see a very proud mother of two and grandmother of five beautiful grandchildren, who I love dearly and who give me enormous joy. I see a retiree who has earnt the right to live life at a slower place doing whatever I choose on any given day. I hope to develop many more personality lines as I settle into this stage of life with, of course, the love and support of my amazing family.

— Ann, sixty-seven, retired Bank Manager (Lise's mother-in-law)

When I was in my teens and twenties, I had such low self-esteem. I think it stems from a dickhead for a father ... but that's a story for another time. I've always had these lines to the side of my eyes when I smile. Always. A guy at a pub once pointed them out and asked how I had crow's feet already. Another dickhead. It stayed with me – I bought eye creams for a while. Cut to my now ex-husband. Again, those lines were critiqued, along with forehead lines, pigmentation from pregnancies, a small top lip – you get the gist. There was a list. It didn't stop at my face.

I spent years fixated on these 'flaws'. I hated looking in the mirror because that's all I could see, and the sadness in my eyes, which I did my best to hide by smiling a lot, creating deeper lines – a vicious cycle.

Now, as a single, empowered, take-very-little-shit, forty-year-old, I will never again allow other people's opinions of me to affect the way I view myself. I have lost so much time. I have wasted time feeling less than. I have been through a lot and I see my lines as experience. With the pain somewhat lifted, my face today looks more youthful. I think stress, deep sadness, and unhappiness made it all appear worse.

I feel stronger every day. I no longer fixate on my so-called flaws every time I look in the mirror. I have a way to go but now I think I don't look half bad. No chance of being mistaken for a thirty-year-old but that's okay. I have two beautiful boys who have quite a few of my features. I look at them and see my mouth, my nose, my crinkly eyes when they laugh, and I think they are beautiful creatures, so how on earth can I continue to see myself as anything but that?

Am I ageing? Absolutely. Do I feel okay about it? Not always. I still feel twenty. I just wish I could go back and shake my twenty-year-old self and tell her to flaunt it. She was fire! So, yes – I'm okay. I'm not fire – more of an ember – and I'm happy enough with that.

— Alicia, forty, Marketing Executive

Until about ten years ago (before kids!), I truly felt like I was looking the best version of myself. I see photos of that woman frequently as I travelled a lot before kids and Facebook memories pop up regularly. Sometimes I feel like I haven't changed much … until I notice my hair is now really grey. I made a deliberate decision to colour it less, but still think of myself as a dark blonde, so it's a bit of a shock when I really look *at myself in the mirror to see that no, that's actually grey!*

I don't like seeing wrinkles, but I know I'd never take serious measures to do anything about them.

I find it amazing how many transformations my body has gone through with four pregnancies. I look at my stomach with amazement at how it grew and shrank repeatedly without any permanent reminders of how large it once was!

Menopause, however, is another story. I wasn't prepared for the weight gain, and I resent the fact I'm looking after myself now better than ever, yet I've gained weight and can't seem to shift it.

Am I scared of ageing physically? Yes and no. I accept its inevitability and the older I get, the more I feel it's a privilege to be where I am. I've never understood why people don't like to disclose their age.

I feel young at heart still – seriously it feels like only a couple of years since I was at uni – so I try not to take too much notice of the woman I see in the mirror who is clearly middle aged!

— Heidi, forty-eight, Physiotherapist

Sometimes I feel like I'd like to shake the young women of today to rise up and protest. There was a whole feminist movement in my era to FREE *women from society's constraints, but this generation is more controlled than ever before. You may be educated and in the workforce, doing some very interesting jobs, but you've lost out in so many other ways.*

To add to this extra burden on women, they are treated as sex objects more than ever. The Barbie image is still very much alive! It's a huge money-making racket to dupe women into thinking they have to stay young-looking forever, exercising themselves to death and buying in on numerous beautifying technologies.

There is a distorted view of how women should age. You are the target audience for so much spin. Men can become 'silver foxes' but women must fight to stay young. It's ridiculous. And it doesn't work either! Even the loveliest of faces gets ruined by too much unnatural intervention. It loses its expression. Work on cultivating your personality and interests, rather than focusing on how you look. An interesting, smiley person will always win out long term over a stiff-faced bore. I once heard two retired top British models who were visiting Australia respond to the question of how to age well. They both said to SMILE OFTEN, *as with every smile your wrinkles disappear into a wonderful expression that defies age. I've always remembered that.*

On the subject of men, there does come a time when as a female you realise that you no longer exude a great attraction to them. Still, by the time that happens, the thought of having to deal with another man and keeping them happy is no longer as desirable as it used to be either. It's a well-known fact that men remarry far more often than women do.

I have, however, always been keen on staying fashionable with clothing and hairstyle, no matter what my age. It's a matter of pride, rather than trying to be super attractive to others. One should always make the best of oneself. Now in my sixties, I get very frustrated with how hard it is to find great clothes for my age group. Those that are can be very expensive. You need to choose more carefully for flattering looks. Men always look so much better because their clothes are more tailored in their cut. I can still make my husband look great at seventy-plus by the clothes I choose for him. (Yes, I've always chosen his clothes!)

When I look at myself now in my late sixties, my biggest regret is my sun-damaged skin, which started showing itself probably in my mid fifties. I didn't notice anything really in my forties, but then I didn't really look for ageing signs at all. My generation lived in the sun without block-out as children and baked for hours sun-tanning in the seventies. I'm certainly paying the price for that now and am prepared to see dermatologists to help with that. I am very hopeful for my daughters and grandchildren, though, that their skins will not suffer the same fate.

Actually, it's looking at my daughters and grandchildren that keeps me happy and content with my life and ageing. I see my lovely and carefree younger self in them so very often. Mind you, I would like them to have MY era to grow up in as females, rather than the current environment. We really did have it good.

— Beryl, sixty-five, Retired Teacher (Sarah's mother)

That depends on how I actually feel! A couple of years ago now, I took on a mindfulness practice to start looking in the mirror and really looking at yourself, seeing what emotion or feeling your face and body show you. It is not about wrinkles or white hair but more about, 'you look really energetic today', or 'at peace', or 'irritated', and leaning into that. It is so wonderful to look into your own eyes and see that sparkle of anticipation, or even the weight of worry, and accepting that feeling. Instead of looking in disgust and saying to yourself 'you look old and need to get to a hairdresser before others see so many white hairs', the new script is, 'you look tired – perhaps the hairdresser is good self-care for you now'. It is not a perfect practice, and of course I have those days where I stare at my cellulite, or style to cover my white patch of hair, but it does help.

The wrinkles and white hair, yep they are there but at forty-three, I've never felt more comfortable in my body. I've wasted many years thinking I needed to look and dress a certain way – the corporate outfits, school mum outfits, the gym outfits …

the list goes on. It was tiring and expensive and I received no validation for my efforts. There was no gushing about my hair or outfits; not because I looked bad, but mostly because I did not feel confident in myself or who I was. This dress-up game then became deeper, thinking I needed to be a different person, losing sight of who I was and what I believed in. I don't know my colour wheel, I don't follow fashion, but I do know myself. I love a fake tan and smoky eye, I love rainbows, glittery eyeshadow, lots of jewellery and leggings are a staple. I may have all of these things on at once, but I feel happy about it, more positive and free to be myself.

And I am not scared of ageing physically. I am scared of Botox, fillers, chemical peels and anything with 'abrasion' in its title. I am scared, actually terrified, of putting chemicals on my skin and in my body after cancer at thirty-two, so I do all I can to reduce my toxic load in the hope it won't happen again. My wrinkles, white hair and saggy skin are all natural, and all me.

— Beth, forty-three, Communications Consultant
and Yoga Teacher

I'll never forget the day I first peered in the mirror (and peered again even closer) at a chin line, so reminiscent of the way my mother's face had aged. I was shocked. My face, this thing I had taken for granted that had largely stayed the same into my early forties, was now changing. And from then, about forty-three, the changes continued with growing speed. But here's the thing – once I got over the initial shock that the girl I had been was slipping away, what grew inside me was a realisation that I had total freedom to decide who this new woman would be. So now, about to farewell a decade of incredible growth, I am the closest I have ever been to the woman I want to be – not pushed and pulled by others' expectations and demands – but aligned to MY *loves and* MY *values. And that is now what I see in the mirror.*

— Nadeena, forty-nine, Communications Executive
and Non-Executive Director

When I look in the mirror I see different things on different days. After an exciting experience, a challenging exercise session or a fulfilling conversation with a loved one, I see a strong and content woman who leads a joyful, privileged life. Other days, when I'm feeling unproductive or irritated, I may notice some jowls that I'm sure weren't there yesterday. But most days I just see me; a healthy, highly functioning forty-year-old who is happy to be alive – fine lines and all. I feel loved by my family and friends and know that my physical appearance does not bother them, so why should it bother me?

— Emma, forty, Chief Financial Officer

How do I feel when I look in the mirror and see my 54-year-old face – well … surprised. I wonder how I got to this age so quickly (and worry that I will find myself at age sixty even quicker!). It is also very sobering to know that the only way I'll ever have youth or young associated with my name now is either through a job with 'youth/young' in the title, or in comparison to someone who is eighty years old.

Am I scared of ageing? Sure. I mind seeing more lines on my face and white in my hair. Sure, I didn't appreciate it when someone doing my makeup asked me to smile broadly so she could get make up into the cracks around my mouth (!) or when the optometrist said as a result of ageing I'd need reading glasses. Sure, it is not fun noticing that, like birds flying south for the winter, so is my skin ... and it isn't just in the winter either that things migrate south on me.

BUT, when I really think about it, I'm probably more worried about my mind and body ageing or failing. And that puts a few things into perspective. I need to work on keeping my body, mind and attitude young and worry about the rest later.

— Rebecca, fifty-four, former Youth Justice Officer

I've never answered a question like this before and my answer surprised me: I feel good when I look in the mirror.

I feel strong, healthy and happy. I don't even notice signs of ageing – maybe that's because I now need glasses! (You see there are positives of hitting mid forties!) Of course, I have days where I feel crap, and look it too, but getting older is not the reason. I've learnt to be kinder to myself on those days.

I've never used expensive creams and until recently never did more than a simple cleanse and moisturise.

Don't get me wrong, I love to 'glam up' for a night out, but that's been the same feeling no matter what age I've been. I have recently started to add a serum to my face but that was because my skin has become so dry due to menopause – another 'bonus' at this age!

I'm not scared of ageing physically in any way. This probably comes from losing two beautiful friends in their early forties to cancer. It has certainly taught me to embrace every day and I know it's a cliché, but I am so grateful to be here, wrinkles and all.

— Violet, forty-six, At-home Parent

There hasn't been a time in my life when I've cared less about what I look like or what other people think of me. That's not to say I don't care about how I look. I do. But I put nowhere near the time and effort into my appearance that I have for most of my adult life and I couldn't be happier.

When I look in the mirror, I see what many 48-year-old women do: wrinkles around the eyes, smile lines, the emergence of age spots, and an increasing number of grey hairs congregating around my temples despite my regular salon visits. But that's about the extent of my self-criticism. On most days, I like what I see.

It wasn't a conscious decision to stop focusing so heavily on what others saw. I think being a full-time working mother meant I simply didn't have the time to obsess over it. Then, as I got older, I realised no one besides me actually cares what I look like (except for maybe my husband and my tweenage daughter). I've never had Botox or fillers and I can't even recall the last time I had a facial. I despise selfies and I've never applied a filter to a photo of myself.

What has been a conscious decision is shifting my life priorities from how I look to how I feel. Over the past fifteen years, I've ticked off a good number of life's most stressful events. I got divorced and remarried, underwent years of IVF, had a baby at thirty-eight then almost died from a post-partum haemorrhage, faced some excruciating challenges in my marriage and with parenthood, and was appointed to a senior management position in my job at a global company. Thankfully, the only negative impact on my health during that time was a recent years-long bout of insomnia, mostly caused by work stress – but I know now that I'm lucky to have emerged so unscathed, both physically and mentally.

It's for those reasons I'm no longer willing to compromise my health for anything or anyone. Over the past eighteen months, I've exercised more than at any other time in the past thirty years and I feel incredible for it. Now I value my physical fitness more than I ever did my wardrobe, my social calendar or my appearance, and it's given me a level of clarity I've never had before around what's really important in my life.

I'm also acutely aware of how my life priorities impact my ten-year-old daughter. I don't want her believing that society only values the genetically blessed or that her success is tied to her physical attributes. I want her to understand that being kind, compassionate and true to herself will make her a strong and successful woman, and it's my job to show her how.

There have been some adjustments. I no longer get the type of attention from men that I used to when I was younger, but I simply don't care anymore. In fact, it's quite liberating. There's a freedom that comes with casting aside the ego and the façade, and with being a no one to everybody except those who are actually important in my life. The only person I want paying me attention is my husband, and fortunately he does (a little too much sometimes).

My paternal grandfather was a hundred and one when he died and my grandmother was ninety-eight. I plan on living just as long but I won't be doing it in front of a mirror. There is too much joy in life to experience.

— Annika, forty-eight, Head of
Communications and Company Director

Saving face

Sarah

It happens gradually, but at some point you'll look in the mirror and see the neon signs of age flashing. Not because you've purchased one of those magnifying mirrors with LED lights from the chemist, but because it is the pay-off for the privilege of still breathing on Earth – and lord knows this is preferential to becoming ashes and dust.

None of this, though, negates the fact it can be confronting to see a *new-you-on-the-way-to-old-you* emerging. My cheeks (all four) are starting to sag. The veins on my hands are positively wormy. My decolletage has sun damage, and it takes at least twenty minutes to de-crinkle after a solid night's sleep. There's a bulging forehead vein the facial equivalent of the Great Dividing Range tracking from smack-bang under my widow's peak to the start of my right brow, it rears with any kind of exertion; whether it's laughing or crying, yelling, or trying to do the Nutbush in heels. It's due to skin becoming thinner and simply another gift of age, but I've grown to appreciate its aggressive presence.

I really like my face; I do. However, with an open-palmed admission, some of the neon lights on it have made me quite self-conscious at times.

At around thirty-four, I began to notice pigmentation spots on my cheeks. At first it was a couple, easily hidden with concealer, but over the following years more began to join up like a patchwork quilt and form larger blotches – an unwelcome surprise thanks to classic sun exposure in youth rising to the surface, and best throw in some post-pregnancy hormones to boot.

Also worth noting, as the owner of skin so pale it would make a cadaver jealous, they were becoming more and more noticeable, which in turn meant more and more foundation to conceal them. In the back of my head was a memory of Mum saying, 'Women should wear *less* makeup as they age' – and here was me at thirty-six basically slapping full-coverage paint on my mug like a pantomime character.

It was time to do something about it.

For me, IPL (intense pulsed light) was the answer. Thanks to the fact laser loves a contrast between light and dark, it meant having gecko skin was a huge benefit, and worked spectacularly well and I was able to throw the thick foundation away.

Approaching my forties, this experience also highlighted the importance of moving skincare to another level. Even though my SPF-game was strong, it had been plain ol' soap and water since youth. The honeymoon was over, baby girl.

My bathroom cabinet is not full of cleansers and moisturisers with 'active ingredients', and retinol, vitamin C, and hyaluronic acid (not to be confused with *hydrochloric* acid – which I did request once) serums are a staple. I'll occasionally book in for a facial and skin treatment.

How my generation of women tackles skincare is so vastly different from that of our mothers – and I occasionally feel a tad self-indulgent when talking to Mum about her own experiences ... or lack thereof. At sixty-six, she's never had a facial in her life, so I picked up the phone to have a chat about it.

Me: Why have you never had a facial?
Mum: They were never available, and only very well-
                to-do women would get things like that done. It

	wasn't ever a focus for me or any of my friends.
Me:	Right. But if you could have got a facial, would you?
Mum:	No! I was never interested in any of it. Nor were any of my friends; we had other things to focus on. And I like my face as it is, thank you very much. Although I do recall women who would go to the hairdresser's once a week.
Me:	Aha! Well, I would never be interested in paying for a blow dry every week.
Mum:	No, it wasn't a blow dry – that concept didn't exist. It was getting your hair set, and then it would last a full week. I do remember that being a thing, but never did it either. [wistful sigh] It was so much simpler back in my day.

See? We're playing on a completely different level with Baby Boomers and beyond. You can't even compare it. And maybe it was better – your face was just your face, and when *nobody* around you was doing anything beyond the bare basics (that is, makeup and Oil of Ulan) with theirs – you were all in the same boat.

....

Sidebar: Isn't it intriguing how our generation is so secretive about having 'work' done, which then differs vastly again with younger Millennials and Gen Z – who appear to have no qualms about changing their looks?

....

Once, backstage at an event Lise and I were emceeing, the 24-year-old event manager was gently touching her lips and quietly chatting with a colleague about how they'd settled down. Our big

I'm happy. As I am right now. This body, this skin, this dry hair with the grey – all of this has gotten me here.

— Urzila Carlson

ears flapping, we interrupted and asked what she was talking about, whereby she promptly pulled out her phone to show us before and after pictures.

We were shocked, and absolutely not because of her newly inflated lips ...

Lise: Hang on, you actually want people to know
             you've had filler?
Her: Hell yes!
Me: Why?
Her: If I've paid $750 to feel better about my mouth,
             then I want people to notice!

What unapologetic freedom to tell her truth.

Because let's be honest, it helps absolutely no one by lying about it – a slow internal reckoning I've come to agree with; pushed over the edge by *another* furphy from a huge Hollywood name in her fifties who regularly insists her completely wrinkle-free visage is solely thanks to sunscreen and water.

Maybe the transition is trickier for women known for their physical beauty – who've had a youth where society held them on a pedestal for looks alone. Perhaps it's self-preservation to fib in order to uphold the ideal of themselves in their own minds, too. I don't have the answer here, but it is yet another middle-aged revelation: what you choose to do or *not* do to your face is nobody else's business but yours.

I love getting old. I have no issues with getting older. I am pumping my face full of Botox – I have no issue with that. I've had lipo, I've had fat-freezing, I've done all of that stuff and that's for me – it's not for anyone else. For me. And I just think it gets better. I have more fun. I'd hate to go back to 22-year-old me fumbling around, not sure about things, going on bad dates. No way. Forty-seven rocks!'

— Shelly Horton

I actually don't have any problem with women doing whatever they need to do to feel good about themselves. If that means that they want to do Botox or fillers or facelifts or whatever, I have no problem with that because I understand the place and the pressure of why they would. If they look in the mirror and they feel better about themselves, so be it.

What I don't love is when women do that and then they say that they haven't done it. I don't like that. I don't like the dishonesty because if you're going to do it, own it. I mean, Dolly Parton talks about how she's more plastic than anything, and I love that. It's so refreshing. Just own it if you're going to do it.

The lie about women not being beautiful is the lie women are not as important as they were when they were younger because they were prettier or they looked better in a swimsuit. We have so much to offer as we get older because of our life experience. We need women forty and over to own who they are and just step into that place of being the wise women who can assist younger women. It can show how beautiful age really actually is.

— Alison Brahe-Daddo

Anti-ageing is just such a horrible term, because ageing is what happens with time – we should be pro-ageing and embracing every new step. Our whole culture is surrounded by youth and beauty and fertility, whereas in other cultures it's the complete opposite: you admire wisdom and elders. We've got a massive job to change that whole mindset, haven't we? Just how that is going to happen in our culture, I've got no idea, but I do think it's important because we can't possibly be expected to look forty when you're sixty, in the same way you can't possibly expect to look ten when you're twenty. It's just not what happens, and as soon as you get your head around that, I think it is easier to live with.

— Dr Naomi Potter

I spy with my little eye

Lise

I'm at war with my pillow. A battle so covert I didn't realise it was happening until it hit me in the face.

To be more specific, the eye.

I've been a side sleeper for four decades, the obsession really setting in during pregnancy when my knees and swollen abdomen made sweet love to a body pillow from Bubs n Grubs. The habit stuck well past my breeding years, and these days even a Jamie Dornan/ Bradley Cooper hybrid would be hard-pressed rolling me out of my right side-sleeping trench. But now, out of nowhere, just for fun, my body has decided to punish me for favouring my right-side ad infinitum.

Welcome to forty, Lise. You are now morphing into a Cyclops.

In Greek mythology, *Kuklops* (Cyclops) means 'round-eyed'. And that's precisely what I see staring back at me in the mirror. One very round left eye, and one teeny, squinty piss-hole-in-the-snow weakling of a right eye.

My facialist friend, Sam, confirmed my pillow theory.

'Oh, for sure. It's called soft tissue atrophy. The bouncy collagen in your face has left the building, mate, so that pillow you're sleeping on? It may as well be a mammogram machine, squashing the flesh from cheekbone to brow bone into oblivion. You're essentially sandwich-pressing the right side of your face.'

Another friend in the beauty industry revealed that some of her very dedicated middle-aged clients rotate themselves through the night like rotisserie chooks from Coles, just to avoid pillow trauma. Others will chock themselves up with different sized cushions strategically placed beneath each scapula, forcing themselves into a Nosferatu-like back-sleeping hell.

I was a bed-wetter when I was younger – perhaps I could track down one of those alarm sheets that trigger when I roll to the right? I'm already using a silk eye mask and have pleaded with Sarah to give me her silk pillowcase. She's six months younger – I'm the emergency right now. Each night I retire to the bedroom, resolutely refusing my right side, only to wake up in the morning, my ocular orbit 0.2 millimetres smaller than the night before.

So, what happens now? Filler and Botox will do the trick, I'm told. A needle stuck straight into the A-frame of my upper eyelid. Opt for this kind of treatment and you may have to contend with droopy eyelids, sagging of the lower lid and difficulty blinking, but at least I'd move out of Greek mythology monster territory, right? All of that to counteract facial volume loss from … sleeping? I am incensed.

My French auntie once told me all about facial massage. I remember being ten years old, watching on as she demonstrated the anti-ageing technique that stimulates pressure points of the face and neck. She'd been to some Vichy spa in the south of France and learned how to manipulate her mug to promote rejuvenated, lifted tissue. There was a lot of cupping, folding, knuckle kneading, tapping and pinching involved. I remember my sister and I stifling giggles as Françoise manhandled her jowls like a Nigella Lawson sourdough.

But maybe she was onto something. If not massage, is there a Romanian dead-lift equivalent for my right eye? Some muscle strengthening exercises I can perform daily to help regain symmetrical, doe-eyed Bambi status? Because right now my peeper is on the receiving end of Thumper's relentless hind foot beating, and I swear to God I'm about ready for wabbit season.

Short of sleeping in a bed pan of hyaluronic acid serum, the reality is that this is perfectly normal. Remember the back-of-the-hand pinch test we'd make our mums do back in the day? Oh, how smug we were, delighting at our taut and juicy skin snapping back into place, while our poor mothers stared on in horror at the pitched flesh-tents just south of their knuckles. Well, it's our turn now. It just is.

So, for the next little while I'm going to raise the white flag and get over myself. I'll probably continue with the chook-on-a-spit technique, and swift upward massage strokes, but that'll have to do, I think.

Yours in ageing asymmetry and Posturepedic pillow warfare,

— Cyclops

....

Update: A few months after writing this, Sarah and I had a work-related photoshoot. As we were going through the proofs with the photographer, it became quite evident to all of us that my teeny tiny right eye was not a figment of my imagination at all. Panic rising, I made an appointment with my doctor to see if medical intervention could provide some options. The doc took one look at me, sent me straight to the optometrist around the corner, who would later confirm it was viral conjunctivitis. Pink eye, guys. Six months of over-the-counter drops to clear it up. The good news? Goodbye nocturnal rotisserie chicken. Hello, sweet right side. Oh, how I've missed you!

....

Fifty shades of (going) grey

Sarah

One of my best friends, Nadsy, has hair so luscious I could almost cry when she effortlessly whips it up into a topknot resembling a red-carpet-worthy coiffure as opposed to my tight, spindly little attempt. (Need a visual? Imagine Severus Snape scraping his hair into a man-bun. Or perhaps Miss Trunchbull when she hammer-throws Amanda Tripp over the fence by her *thick* blonde plaits – which, in hindsight, was perhaps a follicular trigger for nasty ol' Agatha.)

In my forties, I have finally come to accept my fine hair and know it's futile to try to emulate Nadsy's crowning glory, thus retiring my teasing comb. The biggest advantage I can muster is being able to dry my hair in three minutes as opposed to her three days.

We've known each other through the thick and thin of hairstyles, including when Nadsy chopped hers off, dyed it red and channelled *Drop Dead Fred* for a solid six months. There was also her blackest-black fringed bob that looked a bit like a Stackhat. Plus a long chestnut-brown barrel-curl phase. Oh, and a period of rocking scalp-bleaching peroxide white to make Roxette/Pink jealous.

....

Sidebar: I have both hard copy and digital photos of the *D.D. Fred* era, which is why we must stay friends. Although she also has pictorial evidence from when I cut my own fringe with nail scissors, so all's fair in love and friendship-war.

....

Nadsy's type of hair made any style and cut look good, and she'd regularly be stopped by strangers who would *ooh* and *ahh* over it. And, at forty-nine, she's bloody trumped me again ... by going grey. What I thought was utterly fabulous hair in the past is *nothing* compared to the magnificent silver mane she now sports. However, getting there required patience and perseverance – and a big, big wake-up call known as 'The Stripe'.

'The day before leaving for overseas I paid $350 for my monthly balayage, hoping it would last the holiday,' Nadsy said. 'But ten days into the trip, my son took a photo of me sitting across from him and it was a lovely photo – until I saw the grey stripe. I was like, "I am NOT getting away with this anymore. I am THAT lady with a grey stripe, and if I *have* to choose between that and whatever the result, I'll choose grey hair."'

Then forty-six, Nadsy began the journey from 'bronde' (brown/blonde) to her new natural colour – a two-year-long process involving myriad phases.

'Look, I was probably in denial for at least three years beforehand because my appointments changed from every six weeks, to five, then to four,' she said. 'There was a period of should I or shouldn't I with my hairdresser, who admittedly was making so much money from my desperate attempts to hide *the stripe* it's not surprising he erred to *shouldn't*.'

But still, she persisted, letting her regrowth creep out for a couple of months to see what shade of grey she'd been dealt, and committed to the transition. This meant having frank and honest conversations with her hairdresser, who imparted how difficult the first few months would be – and he was right.

According to Nadsy, getting through the first three appointments was miserable, given the most to be done was streaking to blend out the existing dyeline to match her new grey tones.

'It was learning to live with the change, including having conversations – sometimes with completely random people – to explain and justify my decision to stop colouring my hair in my forties,' she explained. 'And I think that when you first start, people see exactly what they are afraid of, which is grey roots and streaks that are *kind of* doing the job you want.

'And while I have always loved the experience of visiting expensive salons, the final few years were such peak maintenance that the mere thought of rescheduling an appointment by even five days would almost send me into a panic of "I can't leave the house with this hair!"'

After a year, hair compliments again began to flow: 'You're so brave!' 'It looks amazing!' 'I could never do what you've done!' And, blowing a metaphorical raspberry to the notion women should get a shorter 'do as they grow older, Nadsy's grey hair cascades halfway down her back, all one length, and parted in the middle in the absolute power-move of middle-aged hair.

In her younger years, Nadsy lived in the pressure cooker that is juggling high-level corporate life as a single parent with full custody.

'I had to be both mum and dad, plus the sole earner, and there were a lot of years lived in masculine *yang* territory so, even though I'm not a girly woman, I did lose my femininity. Only now do I feel I've moved back into my *yin* flow – and my long hair has become a key part of my older identity.'

Furthermore, never again having to factor in hair angst, time, and money – she saved $5000 on salon visits in the first year alone – has been a gamechanger, and on a profound emotional level, too.

'Only now do I feel more like my twelve-year-old self than ever before in my life.'

This stopped me in my tracks, and I had to ask Nadsy what she meant.

'Well, at nearly fifty, I'm through menopause and off the hormonal rollercoaster that started with puberty, my son is a grown man, I stopped drinking, lost weight, and have now let my hair be its natural self. There's a level of security and calm in my life where I do not need to put on a costume that weighs me down – it is absolute freedom.'

Truly, her crowning glory.

Maria's story

Lise

My friend Maria is a powerhouse. We went to high school together from 1993 to 1997. She was vice college captain, a fierce debater, a threat in the pool, a keen member of the choir, and involved in every possible committee, from Amnesty International to theatre sports. She was bold and confident, with a laugh so hearty every student and staff member knew exactly who she was.

We've always kept in touch, so when I saw she'd posted to social media about going to 'normal people gyms' – how she'd often felt she needed to be the right dress size before walking through the doors of certain fitness clubs – I knew it was a conversation I wanted to have with my friend.

In her forties, Maria is stepping into a whole new version of herself. Perhaps you'll see yourself in my friend. Maybe someone you love shares a similar history. This is one account of a woman's determination to change the narrative of her middle years:

I've always been overweight, even as a child. I saw my first dietician at seven and remained a fussy eater until adulthood. I survived on anything white or yellow: toast, chicken nuggets, fish fingers, Maggi noodles and Twisties.

My life has been marked by my weight or size at every age. In grade three, I was weighed in front of my class – 44 kilograms at nine years old. Size 12 at twelve and 65 kilograms, I lost weight for my semi-formal to be a size 16 at sixteen.

As a child she did competitive swimming and, despite the numbers on the scale, knew she was strong. Maria chose to focus on her powerful arms, her whip-smart brain, her infectious laugh and beaming smile:

I was a smart kid, and my smile and laugh always attracted compliments. Some of these were backhanded: 'you could be so beautiful if you lost weight' – I ignored that and would tell people I was beautiful just as I was. While I didn't always believe it, I was stubborn enough to know I didn't want others to tell me how to feel. I don't know where this inner confidence came from!

In her early teens Maria fell in love with fashion. Just like every other adolescent, she desperately wanted to fit in and wear the trends. She saved up her pocket money to buy the iconic Sportsgirl logo tee of the nineties. When the shirt no longer fit, she settled for the branded canvas bag instead:

I had the usual teenage angst: 'if only I was skinnier' to get picked for the fashion parade, or pash a boy at the school dance. 'I hate my thighs!' (even now they are still the biggest part of my body). I come from a long line of pear-shaped women, complete with thunder thighs. Perspective is so important – rather than hating them, I look to it as a connection to my forebears and a link to the strength of country women who raised kids during the Depression. In my twenties, I realised the strength of this. Instead of hating my legs, I realised that my legs keep me standing up, they get me where I need to go and are the perfect spot for my godchildren to sit on and read a book.

On her twenty-fifth birthday, Maria had organised a killer outfit and a nice dinner with friends. She felt amazing ... until she saw the photos. Now a size 26 and 144 kilograms, Maria was at her biggest weight yet. It was then she decided to get serious about food and exercise, shedding 50 kilograms over the next two years. Eventually, life got in the way. She fell in love, began her masters, days were hectic, and she gained the weight back:

As I got older, my lack of fitness and inability to do things started to affect my view of myself. I was so big, I would research restaurants and pick ones with chairs I knew would hold me, I bought business class tickets when I travelled or booked off-peak flights so I knew I would have room and bought additional kids' seats at the footy to give myself more space in a crowded stadium. While I loved me and who I was, my weight was limiting me living my life to the full.

It all came to a head when a fertility doctor delivered the news that Maria's weight was preventing her from conceiving and fulfilling her dream of becoming a mother. Aged thirty-four, she immediately investigated weight-loss surgery, but lacked the family support to undergo that kind of medical intervention. She tried to lose weight naturally, dropped a few kilos, but it wasn't enough.

Two years later, and now thirty-six years old, Maria lost her mum to a sudden heart attack. Her mother's death made her realise how short life was, and at 171.9 kilograms, she began the process for gastric bypass surgery:

I decided to take action, inspired by my younger self who would have done anything to lose weight. To show my commitment to change, I had to lose 20 kilograms before doctors would operate, given I was 'super-size' (their description).

I was busting out of my size 26 clothes and would have to start buying clothes from the United States if I got any bigger. This was about changing a lifetime of poor habits, so I assembled a team of experts: my amazing surgeon, a dietician, and a food psychologist. As time went on, I started following some great social media accounts and bloggers on the same journey and added the gym and personal trainers to my support team.

Now four years since the bypass surgery, 41-year-old Maria has lost 76 kilograms and is a size 12 on top, 16 on the bottom. She knows weight is just a number and says she'd rather focus on improvements in her health and fitness.

The excess skin from her significant weight loss caused bruising and pain, so after enduring repeated skin infections, Maria had a lower body lift to remove 7 kilograms of excess skin. It was one of the hardest things she's ever done, physically and mentally:

In the last few years, I've rediscovered the passions of a younger Maria – small group workouts in the gym discovering my strength, going to concerts without needing a seat, becoming a swimwear confidence ambassador, and discovering national parks when travelling.

I felt like even though I was confident with my body, having surgery was saying differently. It was one of the reasons I opened up about having this 'plastic' surgery. No longer do I have to have a constantly infected belly, or bruises under my arms where I had so much skin.

When I started exercising again, there was no skin needing to be compressed in long compression pants, so my belly didn't hit my boobs, and my arms no longer clapped me as I worked out. I felt free! Surgery made exercising so much easier.

Maria says she still occasionally has insecurities when she's doing something new (who doesn't, right?), but they no longer involve her body:

My worries are more about if I've made the right decisions about relationships, work, or what the future holds. My body has been my constant friend, always there for me – and if I treat it nicely and with love, it allows me to do things I want to achieve.

What's important is how I treat people, not how the outside of my body appears (but it doesn't hurt to love it whatever it looks like!). This is who I'm meant to be. This is me.

Old mole

Sarah

Two words blared back at me from the screen, and one of them was not pleasant: SENILE ANGIOMAS.

There are friendlier terms for the tiny red moles that have started breeding across my trunk, like 'cherry angiomas'. Why the need to swap out cherry for *senile*? Doesn't that mean a crazy oldie? Turns out, no. It's just an archaic medical term simply meaning a characteristic of old age, which is a smidge better but surely completely unnecessary when one is walking the bridge between whippersnapper to senior.

Anyway, who doesn't like cherries? *No one.* They're healthy, a festive staple, and bring to mind nineties Bonne Bell chapsticks, cherry-flavoured Coke paired with hot chips and gravy, and Warrant yell-singing 'Cherry Pie'.

Cherry angioma even sounds like one of the popular girls from school days: Billabong bodysuits with Sportsgirl corduroy A-line skirts, Doc Martens, entered the local Surf Girl comp – and won, pierced her own bellybutton during Biology ... and it didn't even get infected.

Hypothetical Grade 10 versions of Lise and Sarah

Lise: OMG, Sar! You know hot Ando from the bus?

Sarah: Grade 12 Ando – who smells like Joop, looks like

	Bruce Samazan with an undercut, and fills my dreams every night? Nah, don't know him.
Lise:	You dork! Well, you'll never believe who he was macking onto at Tina's party!
Sarah:	Who?
Lise:	Guess.
Sarah:	You?
Lise:	I wish! Don't think he fancies girls with a back brace.
Sarah:	Belinda Zuccarello?
Lise:	Nup, but she's pretty devo about it, too.
Sarah:	Who?!
Lise:	CHERRY ANGIOMA!
Sarah:	Ugh, my heart. Why is she so perfect! Why couldn't God have made me more like Cherry?!
Lise:	Because God needs you for Tournament of the Minds competitions in Gympie, Sarah.
Sarah:	That's it – I'm asking Mum for Doc Martens for my birthday.
Lise:	Find me a safety pin, ice, and a Bunsen burner. I'll meet you in the lab at Big Lunch.

You can picture it, can't you?

Back to the point: I raised aforementioned medical term with the dermatologist at my annual skin check, and she agreed it's quite abrasive – while laughing. We always have good chats while I lie on the bed in my knickers and she studies every square inch of my body under light and magnification, zapping any harmless age spots with dry ice along the way. (At last visit, I thought I had three on my back because fake tan kept adhering to them – she froze ten off. TEN!)

Anyway, Doc told me senile angiomas markedly increase in number from about forty and are more noticeable in pale skin. (Obviously, my brain clocked the first moment I took five scrolls to reach '1980' in an online survey, and immediately ordered the mole troops to march to my torso and let loose with a spitfire approach.) There's usually also a strong genetic link. *Snap* – Mum has a very healthy sprinkling, too.

Then she said the four words I usually don't appreciate directed at me – but absolutely did, in this instance: 'Just a common mole.'

A beer nut, a basset hound and Botox

Lise and Sarah

In our late thirties, as our collagen began to decrease and wrinkles increase, we got Botox. We hereby raise our hands and admit we got sucked into the pressure and panic to erase the early signs of age.

Writing this book has unearthed all kinds of questions and conversations, and so we found ourselves having an honest, sideways conversation during a one-hour car trip about why and how we were pulled into the societal and marketing vortex that is looking younger. Why we were so uncomfortable telling others we had injected our frown line (technical name: glabella), keeping it a secret from most. Why did we feel like fraudsters, tricking our way to compliments, feeling like we were betraying our peers and our maternal line of women whose very genetics we were trying to change?

To be honest, our frown-discontent coincided with the explosion of seeing our faces more than ever before. (There's a reason the global injectables industry experienced a boom during the COVID-19 pandemic: Zoom calls.) Our radio program segments were often recorded and shared to social media – early morning, bleary-eyed broadcasts to strangers, publicity photographs and marketing materials blared on billboards and buses; crowds of hundreds – even thousands – came to events we hosted. With all this came the unsettling insecurity that we had to look as attractive as possible.

The problem was, we convinced ourselves that meant it was time for cosmetic intervention. And sure – while we have no problem spending money on improving our skin integrity naturally with pumpkin peels, IPL (intense pulsed light) therapy and microneedling, it didn't seem to be enough. Everywhere we turned, 'anti-ageing' messages abounded. And at thirty-eight, it felt like we'd just been deployed into a warzone.

There was an odd juxtaposition of emotion around being injected: excitement to no longer look 'cranky' and 'tired', but an unsettling realisation we were cheating. Not just ourselves, not just the people who love us, but the ancestors whose traits had been passed to us.

And where does it stop? Once the glabella was smooth, our attention fell to our nasolabial folds – the lines that run from your outer nostrils past your lips. (Even the fact we are part of a generation of women who know what the bloody hell *glabella* and *nasolabial folds* are, is telling.) Should we 'fix' them with filler? We held off – neither of us convinced, both of us aware of the slippery slope we were on. One injector told Lise the loss of volume around her temples is known as a 'peanut head'. Another told Sarah her hooded eyelids would almost certainly require an eyelid lift in the future, as her vision would likely be impacted. Pardon? Can you feel the fearmongering?

If we didn't *act soon*, would we be two best friends who looked like a beer nut and a basset hound?

But if we did act, would we just look like two women our age … who'd had injectables? It's easy to spot, and a bit deluded to think otherwise. And just because people never asked if we'd had Botox doesn't mean they couldn't spot the lack of frown.

Truth is, we only ever dabbled with the 'tox'; we were entry-level jabbers – once or twice a year at best. Our brief to the cosmetic nurse –

'super subtle but make it *fresh*', believing the lie we've been sold that ageing faces are, in fact, stale.

You can only keep up with so much. Once you start to focus your energies on every corner and facet of your face – you will see everything. Where does it stop?

It's a clever trick, isn't it, to scare women into thinking they look angry. Daresay, is it an extension of the persistent expectation for women to always look pleasant, friendly and *nice*? 'You'd be so much prettier if you smiled.' How many times did we hear that as young women with faces simply in repose?

Please know, it's without a hint of ego we admit our faces had been considered pretty for most of our adult lives. While we were aware of our looks, and even earned money off them for a while, the level of facial scrutiny we had placed ourselves under as we stood on the precipice of youth and middle age was intense. And each time we left the injector's rooms, we'd feel turmoil and a tinge of sadness, like we'd committed the ultimate treachery against something that had treated us well.

What were we frightened of? Our looks fading? Of heads no longer turning in our direction? We decided to play the tape, 'what would people say if we just let nature play out?' 'She's aged.' Yes, that's factually correct. We are ageing. AND WHAT OF IT?

We want to love our changing faces. We want to trust our bodies, the way our bodies have trusted us, and embrace not erase.

It goes without saying that none of our musings relate to corrective surgery, or those experiencing true anguish and despair when they look in the mirror. Do whatever you need to do to feel better and more confident – and if that's needles or threads, then do it. Life is too short to feel sad and unhappy over things that can be fixed.

But we were just feeling like we *should* do something about a natural process that every. single. person. in. the. world. must navigate as they biologically age. And so many of our counterparts feel the same. We're the first generation to have such a broad range of choices, and it can feel confusing and self-obsessed to be worrying so much about appearances when quite simply, ageing is not an option *when you want to live*.

Society conditions women to believe we *lose* beauty as we age – that it's something that disappears, never to be seen again, like a misplaced sock. The only thing that is lost is youth.

If we're honest, we are constantly seeking faces who haven't succumbed to the pressure. (Again, there is absolutely no judgement for those who do, because we've been there.) Why should choosing *not* to alter ageing features feel like a rebellion? Now we wonder if we can change the script so younger women aren't scared of growing older. Spending time and money seeking the physical characteristics of youth is a fool's game.

For now, we've stepped away from the needles. Perhaps we will feel differently down the track, and, like everyone, we reserve the right to choose. It feels like the right thing to do for us out of respect for all the women who've gone before us, and to provide an option to all the women who come after us.

Relationships

Just because your relationship status changes doesn't mean life isn't going to be still the most exquisite thing, and it's what you make it. There's a saying: 'glass half-empty or glass half-full'. The fact is the glass is refillable – so just fill it up!

— Emily Jade O'Keeffe

A time of reckoning

No one wants to talk to their husband at night! Everyone wants to get their phones and a cup of tea or a glass of wine and pop into bed and watch Bravo Housewives. I don't want to talk to anyone, I'm going to have forty-five minutes to myself, then I'm going to sleep. No one's having FUN. *Gawd.*

— Beth Macdonald

Dating in your late thirties is not like dating in your twenties, men have a lot more baggage – as do women – and I was too old to be let down, I was too old to go through all that again; I felt tired. I'd been through it all a million times.

It's better to be alone than with someone who doesn't value you. For me, I would rather be alone and go to bed every night than be in a relationship where I wasn't happy. Don't be afraid of being on your own.

— Samantha X

It actually sounds like a rom-com and I'm allowed to say that because I went through the cesspit of ten years between marriages, where I thought I'd get snapped up straight away. And strangely enough, I didn't! I dated so many of the wrong guys and had a horrible time. I'd almost resigned myself to the fact that I was going to be single for the rest of my life.

It was soul-crushing doing that dating – like a decade of, 'am I doing this right'? Feeling rejected, just not having that connection, or making the wrong choices. Like, you know, I ended up seeing a guy who was in a relationship thinking he would leave her for me, and now I just feel icky about it. Like, what was I thinking?! I look back at my desperate self and just go, 'you deserved so much better'. And I think, though, part of getting older is you've got to make all of those mistakes so you then go, 'right, here's what I will accept, here's what I won't accept, and here's what I want'.

I think I'm lucky I stumbled into the right bar at the right time, and honestly – it's a life changer.

I tell this story to give people hope, because I'm also the girl who went on an RSVP date with a guy who was missing a front tooth – and still pashed him.

— Shelly Horton

There are certain times in my life where I've been brought to my knees, but I just remember last year, after the separation, going to a friend's house and I tried to get down the driveway and before I could get to her front door, I was actually on my knees. Like, a hot mess; I know what it means to say that now. I think it's because you don't expect to not grow old with the person you thought you would. Nineteen years is a long time. It's taken enormous amounts of courage to come out the other side of that. I mean, gosh, be alone? That scared the bejesus out of me more than anything in my life.

I did say to all my friends, do not set me up with anyone, don't let me ASK *you to set me up with anyone, I'm not going on dating apps, I'm not doing any of those things. Then the first night I was on my own, I got Uber Eats and was like, I'll just have a look on*

Bumble. I'll just see. And sure enough – the first person I swiped is the person I'm still with a few years later. It's extraordinary. A beautiful love story, I must say.

— Taryn Brumfitt

Look, I've dated through the decades and have been able to witness how it's changed over the years, and also I date men of all different ages. So, I will date guys in their twenties through to their fifties, because why not?

Now what is a really interesting phenomenon, what's actually shifted, of course, is technology, but not for the obvious reasons. What it's done more broadly is made us what I call 'smaller humans' – we have lost the resilience of discomfort. We have no ability to sit in the discomfort of, for instance, ringing Mr Wilson and risking that somebody might say no when you ask them out on a date. We have cocooned ourselves from that discomfort via various technological services over the years.

Resilience is a muscle. If we don't prime that muscle, we've got no capacity to actually rise up – and it takes a rising up to ask somebody out on a date; it's called vulnerability, you know. It's hard, but we don't like hard. We don't have to actually sit in our unknowingness or uncertainty or discomfort around anything anymore. We don't even have to wonder how long our pizza is going to take when we order it on an app, because there's a little orb that follows its way through the suburb. It's like, oh good, it's thirty-five seconds away.

So, in the dating realm, I think it comes out to play in probably the most horrible, horrible of ways. We don't know how to do intimacy. Young people today are dating less and less. They're losing their virginity later and later; half of all people under thirty in Japan are virgins and it's because they are so frightened of 'in real-life confrontations'. They are so attuned to being able to communicate in what I call a connection-lite kind of manner online, where you can just send an emoticon when something gets difficult, or you can pretend you didn't see a text when it gets confrontational.

I guess in some ways, I sort of survived by seeing it as a bit of an experiment, and I don't mind being really upfront about this but, so far this year, I have had ten no-shows. I had number ten two weeks ago. Literally, I get texts that go, 'Hey, maybe we should have a coffee someplace, somewhere'. And I say, 'someplace sounds wonderful'. Nobody wants to be the person who's foolish enough to ask for it to be defined.

— Sarah Wilson

This has been through my forties where, having been a mother for so long and having put myself at the bottom of the list, it was this slow reckoning of going, 'wait a minute – I actually have needs' and don't want to be stuck in a specific role like this for the rest of my life. That has been incredibly freeing, and also really challenging to be able to go, 'I'm not going to be cooking dinner, I'm going out to my Pilates class tonight – you guys figure it out'. As I've aged, there's just been so much more permission I've given myself to put myself an equal first.

In the shifting landscape of a marriage, I think there does need to be a lot of discussion, a lot of empathy. In the sense of, as a woman, your priorities do begin to change and I had been putting my husband ahead of me and my needs as well. He then became equal to what I needed – so communication is everything and you can get through it, without a doubt. On the other side of it, I think, is actually a really wonderful, exciting, different, more balanced marriage than perhaps what was there before.

— Alison Brahe-Daddo

Samantha's story

Lise

I met Samantha in the most undignified position a woman can find herself in – 'Happy Baby' pose in a reformer class. For the uninitiated, let me paint a picture. You're flat on your back, the arches of your feet lassoed in straps, legs akimbo, splayed open like a Lycra-clad BBQ chook, as you gently rock from side to side. Not dissimilar to a baboon presenting, really. So, I'm there, outlines of minora and majora in plain view, trying not to make eye contact with anyone, when from the reformer bed beside me I hear a gravelly, 'Well, this is the most action I've gotten in three months!'

Ladies and gents, I give you Samantha.

I knew in that instant she was my person. A sense of humour so bold and unapologetic, Samantha was a big personality in my weekly Pilates class. Booming voice, confidence in spades, cropped hair with a feature faux-hawk – this woman was magnetic.

I told Sarah about her the next day:

Me: 'I've met this woman. She's unreal. I need to be her friend, and I can tell she has a big story to tell.

Sarah: Is she forty? Otherwise, she's no good to us.

Me: That's the kind spirit I know and love. Are you jealous?

Sarah:	It's just that I thought I was the only friend you'd picked up all those years ago. And you've probably lost your friend-date touch, old duck.
Me:	Challenge accepted. I'm asking Samantha out!

At the next class, I nervously sidled up to Samantha and asked how her groin was feeling – you're all free to use that line next time you want to befriend someone – and the rest is history. Samantha and I got to talking and we haven't really stopped.

I'd been right. Samantha is a complex, layered, colourful woman who's lived a life. Her stories about touring Iceland with Def Leppard and Whitesnake as a self-confessed twenty-something groupie are among some of my favourite.

Today, Samantha is a 44-year-old mother to a seven-year-old girl, and proud co-parent. She won't use the term 'ex', despite her marriage of seven years coming to an end in 2019. She says the prefix feels inaccurate when defining the relationship she has with her child's father.

Before I give you the four-one-one on the extraordinary co-parenting life Samantha has designed for herself in her forties, I feel it's important to share some of her story, to really understand what has driven and shaped this woman's decisions and fierce resolve when it comes to her non-conventional familial setup.

Samantha's parents split when she was six years old, her father a transient, unreliable character in her life. She grew up with her younger sister and her mother, and for reasons she still doesn't quite understand, Samantha's mother favoured her sister. With hindsight, Samantha thinks her mother may have suffered from untreated postnatal depression following her birth, combined with many narcissistic traits. Samantha often felt lonely and sidelined, seeking her mother's love but never quite getting it.

> Many of us get wiser as we get older, but not many of us get
> sober as well ... but can I just tell you, sobriety brings with it a
> superpower and clarity like you've never known, you've never
> ever known.
>
> I think if there's one woman in the world you don't
> really want to mess with it, it's probably an alcoholic who's
> recovered in their forties with nothing else to lose ... it's a
> wonderful place to be. I'm just going to tell you point-blank,
> I love being sober!
>
> *— Shanna Whan*

When Samantha was twelve years old, she decided to live with her father, who'd since put down roots with a son he'd had from a previous marriage. Samantha's half-brother was thirteen years her senior, a strapping twenty-five-year-old man who she idolised. He shattered her world when he sexually assaulted her on the couch that had become her temporary bed. Her father blamed her, explaining his son had been lonely, and made Samantha swear not to tell a soul.

Life after that was angry and destructive. Samantha acted up and struggled in school. She got drunk and stoned on her thirteenth birthday, barely passed year twelve, tried university for six months but frequented the bar over the lecture hall every time. Her twenties were spent looking for love in all the wrong places.

'I would take any scrap that was thrown my way. I had no reference of how a man should treat me, as my dad was never around to lay that foundation,' she said. She lived and partied hard.

In June 2010, now in her early thirties, Samantha met Gary at a friend's barbecue. He wasn't her usual type, but that was a good thing. Samantha and Gary's relationship was G-rated for a long while. She was determined to fall for him as a person as opposed to getting swept up in the sexual pheromone storms she'd navigated in the past. The pair were wonderfully in sync and developed a bond deeper than anything she'd ever hoped for. They were engaged in 2011, married in June of 2012 and became parents the following year.

Samantha endured a traumatic birth and was diagnosed with postnatal depression when her baby was nine weeks old. She was hospitalised for three weeks at a private psychiatric unit for mothers with PND.

'It was a long journey getting well but PND was the best thing that ever happened to me. It completely stripped me back to bare bones and I had to rebuild a new me,' she said.

So, Samantha 2.0 made changes as she set about redesigning her new life, starting with her marriage. Her relationship with Gary had been strained from the events following their daughter's birth, but Samantha was determined they stay together as a family. They went to counselling, together and separately.

'We loved each other so much but what we had to give, what we wanted to give, and the way we wanted to give it just didn't match up. We were sacrificing our happiness so our daughter could have her parents together, but we were living a life neither of us wanted.'

It was during counselling that Samantha and Gary uncovered a truth about their relationship that would set them both free. Gary, a 'beautiful man with Asperger-y traits', realised he was asexual – a sexual orientation sometimes defined by the lack of sexual attraction to others, or a low interest in sexual activity. Asexuality can mean different things to different people, but to Gary, the realisation made the puzzle pieces of his life, and marriage, finally fall into place.

Had Samantha known all along? Had she suspected anything of the sort? Did she feel rejection, or relief? She freely admits knowing, from the moment she and Gary met, that they were sexually incompatible. At a cellular level, she knew her connection with him was different. She recalls it being a conscious, considered choice, to forgo an active marital sex life – to 'forfeit the fireworks', in exchange for a man who'd love her unconditionally, the way her family had never been able to.

It took a couple of years for Samantha and Gary to work out what the next chapter of their lives would look like. At forty-two, they officially separated. The decision was to uncouple but remain a family. They hatched a plan to purchase a block of land, with Gary's father building a two-bedroom granny flat for his son and a three-bedroom home for Samantha – a Jack-and-Jill garage connecting the two dwellings so their daughter could move as she pleased between the 'boy house' and the 'girl house'.

Once the construction dust had settled, life became surprisingly uncomplicated and happy. Samantha speaks proudly of her pale pink front door, and the satisfaction she feels from keeping her family unit intact. Weekly burrito nights are spent together, while other evenings Samantha will happily binge Netflix with a glass of pinot gris knowing her daughter is down the hall, across the garage and with her father. An idyllic set-up, unimaginable and likely impractical for most separated couples. Samantha credits communication and the absence of sexual jealousy – a silver lining to the asexual cloud – for the success of their unique arrangement.

She'd been honest with Gary and told him that, eventually, she'd want to explore the dating world, recognising how much she'd missed the romance and physicality of a relationship. Gary agreed and acknowledged this was only normal. Ultimately, he wanted to see Samantha happy. He was fine with it.

In her forty-third year, Samantha downloaded a dating app. Minutes later, she deleted it.

'My confidence was shot to shit, as I'd been in a relationship for nine years where my partner hadn't focused on my looks, clothes, lingerie, Brazilian, no Brazilian. I didn't know where I rated in terms of "hotness" and desirability.' Samantha recalibrated her approach. Her twenty-fifth high school reunion was approaching, so she decided to see if her first love was single. He was.

'I thought, if I'm going to throw my leg over for the first time in a long time, I want it to be with someone I feel comfortable with.' After a few months of texts and phone calls, Samantha flew to Adelaide for 'The Reunion'.

'I thought I had lost my sex drive forever, and this was what life was going to be. Holy guacamole! There was a fire lit under me! It felt so good to be alive and sexual again. Turns out I was still that twenty-year-old turbo!' COVID and distance meant her fling was short lived, but Samantha insists it was 'good to get back in the saddle'.

With restrictions lifted, Samantha felt ready to step into the local dating pool. As a forty-something-year-old woman, she was not prepared for the level of attention she received.

'I used to have the most gorgeous long hair and had to chop it all off following a psoriasis diagnosis. Hence the faux hawk. To be honest, I figured it was the perfect "dickhead shield", given I wasn't interested in meeting anyone that was just into looks.'

Samantha was upfront about not wanting to get married again, not wanting any more children, and not wanting to live with someone. Her boundaries were crystal clear. She set about gamifying her dating.

'I had questions I'd send each suitor. The ones who answered went through to the next round. The ones who didn't were deleted.'

- If you could invite anyone in the world to dinner, who would it be?
- What constitutes a perfect day for you?
- What was the last song you sang along to?

- Is there something you have dreamed of doing for a long time? Why have you not done it?

Samantha never wore makeup on her first dates – a self-imposed protocol.

'I wanted them to take me as I am, plus I wasn't going to put that much effort in for some random I didn't know!' After a couple of weeks on the app, she'd racked up 2875 likes.

'I nearly died! I had 29-year-olds wanting to date me! I went on a couple of dates with those young ones as it was quite the ego stroke, if I'm honest. I remember thinking, "Who is this person?" about myself. The sexy chats, the messaging. It was all so millennial!'

Samantha would often check in with Gary over a morning coffee.

'I asked him if maybe he was interested in dating, and he said he was more interested in the currency of Nigeria!' Exhale. Permission. Acceptance. Whatever you want to call it, Samantha realised it was okay for her to chase her happiness. They were good, her and Gary.

Despite having Gary's full support, Samantha decided to step back from online dating.

'Look, it's a bit of a mind game, and I really like meeting people the old-fashioned way. I had a great time, but it wasn't sustainable going out for drinks and spending too much time getting sucked into swiping.'

For now, Samantha is living her best single life in her pale pink girl house, her daughter and co-parenting partner right beside her, through the garage. As for Pilates class, 'Happy Baby' pose has now become my happy place. You just never know who you'll meet lying on your back and holding your feet.

Bonnie's story

Sarah

Bonnie looks like a main character out of *Vikings*, or at the very least someone you'd want on your side in an apocalypse. We met through mutual friends in our twenties when we were both footloose, fancy-free and living in the same city, and kept in touch over the years. She is savvy, powerful and athletic, a tall and assured woman with a crazy mass of ringlets and smiley green eyes – a physical aura that makes you want to be in her presence. She's quick to laugh – a deep-throated sound almost always accompanied with her head thrown back. She can tell a tale with comic timing that's second to none, and she's the edgy cool girl who has never failed to make me belly laugh over the years. I never, ever in a million years would have guessed she was deeply unhappy in her long-term relationship.

At forty-four, Bonnie finally left Drew, the father of her two young children. The fellow she met and fell in love with sixteen years before at an exercise bootcamp had long since disappeared. Where first he was kind, solid and dependable, over the years he had instead morphed into an angry, financially controlling man who drank too much.

'Drew was a superstar in my eyes when we met,' Bonnie said. 'He lived an exciting lifestyle, everybody knew him; it was another world, and I was enthralled. It's tough to pinpoint when it started to go wrong – it was never a single moment, but rather death by a thousand cuts.'

I've seen so many women who didn't understand what was happening financially – or they split up and presumed they were doing better than they were or their partner had run up debts. And now they've found themselves in their forties not where they thought they should be. This has meant they now had to not only figure out HOW to run finances which they never had to before, but actually had less than they thought because they took their eyes off their finances and left it to their partner. So it's in our best interest to keep our eyes on our money, even if we think we're not great at it.

— *Mel Browne*

In hindsight, she believes their troubles began when they went from separately enjoying high-performing jobs interstate and overseas, to starting a small business together. Suddenly, their lives were downscaled to living and working in one suburb, and overwhelming financial struggles and debt followed. The relationship began to crumble, and neither of them knew how to stop it further deteriorating.

'We endured incredibly stressful times in an intensely localised life, and it eventually broke us apart. My situation involved having no control over any financials – plus I worked in the business without pay for a really long time, so I couldn't leave because I had no money. I just felt enormous pressure to make the relationship work and was horribly embarrassed that I had gotten myself into such a situation.'

The last three years were especially difficult. Bonnie's discontent was growing – and so was the amount of alcohol she was drinking to mask her unhappiness. After discovering she had an ulcerated stomach, Bonnie finally quit.

'I increased the amount of alcohol I was drinking to cope with being miserable, which then made me more miserable – it was a vicious loop. My emotions and drinking were out of control, the finances and paperwork were a clusterfuck of distress, and I wasn't being the parent I wanted to be.

'I can remember looking in the mirror and just being so saddened by what I saw. I was fading away, lost in stress, gaslighting, sorrow, and alcohol. I thought, is this it? FUCK. Is this what we become? Just lifeless shells? I began to see other lifeless middle-aged women walking around too and thought, something has to change.

'I couldn't stay, I really couldn't – but I knew I needed to be sober to be able to leave and have a stable job so I'd be ready to look after the children on my own.'

The fear of being a single mother was nothing for Bonnie compared to the fear of staying in the relationship and never realising her full self again. She began the slow and steady journey to build her self-worth – turning to podcasts and online communities for women who wanted to rediscover their identity.

'In those final years of the relationship, I began re-wilding myself. I cleared out a whole bunch of stored crap, stored trauma from my body. I was able to grieve a pregnancy. I learned what deeply turns me on, after spending years in a relationship where Drew considered my desires inappropriate and too intense. I learned from amazing women about the importance of practising pleasure on a daily basis, and how it's my responsibility to work on my own pleasure – it's a gift to everyone around me if I'm juicy and alive.

'I thought about the example I was setting for my children, how as their mother it's my responsibility to show them – not just tell them – women are all the things: loud, funny, kind, loving, silly, beautiful, well-respected and loved. I couldn't do that as a half a human in an unhappy relationship. My self-worth was solid when it came time to finally leave.'

The tipping point came when Drew was passed out one night and Bonnie picked up his phone.

'It was one of those magical moments where the universe steps in and taps you on the shoulder. For no reason, I picked it up – only to see two intimate messages from a woman. There were no other messages from her that evening that he'd forgotten to delete.'

She discovered Drew had a long-term involvement with the woman, who lived interstate, and had been staying with her during 'work trips' away from Bonnie and the kids.

'I don't blame him for seeking someone else because I would have been tough to live with in those final years as I evolved from being a co-dependent, submissive partner to a woman in her full roar – but the real nail in the coffin was when he lied to my face.

'He looked into my eyes and said he hadn't stayed with her. When I told him I knew otherwise, he said, "I don't have to tell you anything". It was at that moment I realised he had no respect for me, and there was no recovering this relationship. It was time to leave. Their relationship was one of the best things that ever happened to me.'

And so, with the children in tow, she left – and felt nothing but freedom and relief.

Now forty-six, and still in the thick of her life reset, Bonnie knows there is more wisdom and reflection to come. For now, it's a process of treating herself with kindness, and slowing her pace to maintain a healthy nervous system for the children – who now enjoy lives full of laughter, hugs and attention and are no longer being raised in an unhappy, toxic household. Her biggest challenge to date has been learning how to manage her money. It's been a slow process, working through the damage of past control and conditioning to get back up on her feet.

'I think Drew was shocked I had the balls to leave. But, then again, maybe I'm the one who was shocked I had the balls to leave. The system we live in creates the narrative that single mothers aren't that great – and that's bullshit. We are fucking awesome, and what I didn't know was that it could be this good!

'I love my life now with an intensity I had been craving for years. I just bloody love it. I laugh more – so much more. I have my life force back. I take up space in the world. I dance. I smile. I'm more confident. I feel more beautiful – like a glorious, sexual being. I am excited by the future.'

Nowadays, every morning at dawn, Bonnie dives into the ocean and swims – rain, hail, or shine. The self-confessed health fanatic initially began simply to test the fitness benefits of cold-water therapy, but it quickly became so much more.

'It makes me feel exquisitely alive, joyful, childish, and in awe. When I swim with my mates, our rule is to do a massive "whoop!" before we jump in the cold water. We giggle every time.'

Bonnie smiles. 'I'm me! Finally, I'm me again. I am the kind of mum I always wanted to be. I am the kind of woman I was dying to be.'

Jordana's story

Lise

A few years ago, I witnessed bravery, self-love, and will power in action.

Jordana and I met at the local kindergarten when our eldest boys were four. She was beautiful, with her mane of dark hair, kind eyes and broad smile. Her accent was exotic – she was a Brazilian national who'd come to Australia in her twenties, fallen in love with an Australian man, and made a life here. In her late thirties when we first met, she was a tertiary-educated high school teacher who juggled full-time work and suburban family life.

It didn't take long for J and me to connect beyond the obligatory raffle drives and working bees. We both had two sons – our firstborns played toddler tennis together once a week, while the babies sucked on rusks and pine bark at park playdates. We felt comfortable being in one another's homes, having bottomless cups of tea on the living room floor, our bare feet tucked beneath us as we chatted about life, motherhood, marriage and careers.

J is one of those women who refuses to pretend. There is no veneer with her. She began confiding in me about problems at home. Her husband was an alcoholic, and despite trying to keep things under wraps, word was getting out. He'd shown up to kindy inebriated to pick up the children; she'd received a phone call at work, from the centre director. It was not the first time. Her life was complicated and hard. So much harder than anyone could imagine.

The alcohol abuse had bled into every crevice of J's life. She'd become the sole breadwinner because her husband could no longer hold down a job, let alone successfully apply for a new role; she had two small children to protect from the dysfunction; she hardly slept, left to manage his midnight drunken episodes; was still tending to wakeful babies, and then having to get up for work at 5.30 a.m. each morning. When the alcohol wore off, he was paranoid, controlling and manipulative. She knew she had to leave.

J played the tape over and over in her mind: 'If I leave, I will never be able to have what I have now' – a mantra she tortured herself with, and one that kept her rooted in place for longer than it should have.

'The truth is,' she said, 'I'd grown too attached to the house, the big renovation dream we'd had, the idea of a perfect family unit, the joint finances. I was scared of being poor. I got so caught up in those things.'

But things had become unbearable at home. Her eldest son had shown signs of anxiety; not yet five, he knew what was going on. J remembers driving around the suburb alone one day, her body riddled with stress, her knuckles white from gripping the steering wheel so tight.

'I pulled in under a tree to catch my breath, my hands still hurting from how tightly I'd been squeezing. And then, I just let go. I let go of the steering wheel, and it felt like I was floating. And it hit me: Oh my God – nothing in this world belongs to me, anyway! This car is here to serve me, but it's not really mine. The house is there for me to live in, but it doesn't feel like home. I had this moment of clarity and detachment – from the notion of material possession and my worth in all of it. I realised that I was not allowing my life to happen because I was afraid of losing *things*. I'm living in misery because I'm afraid to lose the house in the good suburb. I felt at peace. Maybe it was spiritual, I don't know, but I thought, I can do this. I can actually live and rebuild something else. I do not want to live with an alcoholic anymore.'

J is smart, so smart. She was able to assess her own vulnerability with such objectivity, and she knew the key to her success would be to have the right people in her corner. She'd tried to leave before, staying with friends for short bursts of time, but she'd always gone back. This time, she knew her plan needed to be watertight.

'I surrounded myself with people who weren't just "nice". I needed people to take action for me, and with me. I found a counsellor who guided me through my options. She did the mapping for me – what my departure would look like, the timeline. We created a calendar, a step-by-step plan. That's what I needed because I couldn't even conceive of how, or where to start. By having someone like that, it made me accountable. I can change my mind a lot. I didn't trust myself.

'She'd check in with me: "Are you still strong with this? Are you still confident about this?" She would remind me of why I wanted to leave in moments of uncertainty and weakness.'

A plan of action under her belt, J set about getting ready, quietly, and methodically. Her financial situation in the lead-up was solid, given her full-time employment and her husband's fortunate disinterest in the family's financial situation.

'I prepared for six months. That was the plan. I started saving my money and slowly buying what I would need – kettle, toaster. I locked them away in a cabinet in the garage. It was thrilling, in a way, buying things just for me, things I liked.'

Planning her escape required J to be strategic and clever. Her husband allowed her to be out of the home as long as it was work-related, so with the support of her employer, J started finishing work an hour earlier, making appointments with legal aid, the bank and domestic violence services at the back end of her workday. She would squirrel away time to educate herself on where she stood financially and legally.

'You learn to lie. You enter survival mode. You have to lie, to pretend, when you're dealing with someone toxic. I'd make my appointments, I'd get the information I needed, or I'd see my counsellor. Because it's so hard to do it on your own. That's why women don't leave.'

J tells me about how hard it is step into someone you're not; to act and make decisions you're not used to making. The secrecy and the lying went against her traditional Catholic upbringing. She tells me about the two very important words her counsellor armed her with.

'She told me, "Jordana, you have to be selfish and ruthless. This is not the time to be compassionate. This time you must be selfish and ruthless." It went against everything I was ever told to be, as a woman – servitude, compassion, sacrifice, honest. I had just turned forty when my counsellor gave me this advice. She was in her fifties – and so, because she was older and had been there herself, I knew I could trust her.'

One month out from D-day, J signed the rental papers on a small house and slowly started furnishing it with pre-loved pieces and marketplace finds.

'Nesting gave me so much hope. Sometimes, I'd just drive there after work and spend time in there alone. It was a place where I felt safe. I would exhale and think, "I can't believe this is happening. Soon I'll be free!" I manifested this house for myself. I needed my rent to be under $400 per week. Nobody wanted this place – it had been on the rental market for three months. It was in really bad shape, weeds all over the yard. I took it as it was. I wanted this house. I offered $380 and they accepted.'

When she was forty-one, her boys only three and four, J packed

> I sought it [legal counsel] pretty much straight away. In my first marriage, I walked away because I didn't want to be in it anymore and felt so much guilt about it, I said 'you have everything' and I had to restart again. I didn't want to do that again – I'd worked too hard, and I was really fearful of losing a lot of things.
>
> — *Emily Jade O'Keeffe*

up her car and drove to meet me. It was the first week of the summer holidays, and I'd rented a little unit at the beach. It was just me, J, and our boys. It would give her a momentary pause in what would be the boldest, most daring and defining week of her life. The perfect cover – a palatable story to tell her husband, to explain the packed bags at the door – an ideal circuit-breaker.

We sat on the balcony overlooking the ocean where she told me everything; the plan she'd been working on for half a year and the fact that after our short beach stay, she'd be moving into her new home, and never going back to her old one. I'll never forget the resolve, and sheer exhaustion, etched on her face.

Starting a new life wasn't easy. Nor was shaking the old one. A lot of challenging and traumatic things happened over the next few years. J was hammered with emotional blackmail and relentless threats.

'I realised how under his spell I was. How submissive I'd become. How much he'd manipulated me: "You're going to ruin Christmas! You can't do this!" He knew my weak points. But this time, I held strong.'

She made the decision to cut back from full time work to two days of teaching each week.

'It's what the kids and I needed – to be together. I learned that my family tax benefit would be bigger if my salary was smaller, so I made the decision to drop back while the boys were so small. They'd just lost their family unit; I didn't want them in after-school care all the time while we were navigating this; I wanted to be able to volunteer at school, give them a sense of normality, for them to know that I was right there, to minimise the trauma. My little one started prep but I had to pull him out on the school's advice. He just wasn't coping. He needed to be home with me. I co-hired a nanny with my neighbour – we shared the nanny – so we could both work on the days we had to. I tried to keep life as small and simple as possible for us. But it was a big sacrifice, financially.'

Money was tight but J was resourceful. She was also kind to herself when she needed it.

'I used to be so precious about buying things from op shops – I never liked it. But now I realise how great it is and I love it! One thing I did, though, was spend good money on a brand-new bed. I needed to sleep. I was so tired. I could never sleep properly in my old life. He'd wake me at 3 a.m., drunk and ranty. All I could think was, "I need a good bed!" I went to the bed shop – got measured and scanned by a computer! – all to find the perfect bed just for me. It was so important, this bed purchase – symbolic, even, for the fact you're not going to be sleeping with that person anymore, and it wasn't another hand-me-down. It was all mine.'

Transitioning to a new normal has been challenging for J. She says she still operates in survival mode most days.

'It's just been one foot in front of the other. I look at people around me, growing, doing things, buying houses, progressing. I can't do that right now. My priority is my boys. That's why I've made the choice, for now, to be home with them as much as I can, living on a very small salary. It's just the three of us, so togetherness is my main focus.

If they're happy, then I'm okay. There are many moments of joy, pride and freedom. I look out my kitchen window and I think, "My God, I'm good! I don't have any problems. We're doing fine! Yes, it's hard to do everything on my own and be the only one there for my children, but at the same time I now feel completely in control."'

Today, J has officially been divorced for two years and her boys are twelve and nine. She works as a casual relief teacher three days a week.

'My profession pays well this way. I'm lucky. I'm enjoying being a supply teacher. I had to drop the status around my career and get comfortable with "you're just a relief teacher", but I love it.'

Her home is modest, peaceful, full of love, gorgeously curated in her warm, J way.

'There is a lot of wealth in the area my boys go to school. My eldest son, he's embarrassed to bring people back to our house. And that's so hard for me. Most of his friends come from stable families, with the big houses and the pools and all the things that kids want, because both mum and dad work and earn well. "Mum, you're doing all this by yourself" – he knows; he's realising. But it's still really, really overwhelming for me sometimes. We might not have as much, but my boys feel a lot of freedom to be who they are in our home. We don't watch the news or footy on TV because we don't like it; dinner is casual as the three of us eat like birds; we do a lot of things spontaneously, like going to the beach or watching a movie with popcorn in the middle of the week, just because. It's lovely.'

J admits that life certainly didn't go along the way she'd planned. At forty-seven, her focus is moving from a place of struggle to one of growth and achievement.

'There are so many things I've experienced that I could never have imagined when I was younger. I have learnt so much. I've learnt to recognise red flags in people, and how to quickly notice their real intentions.

'I want to grow. I see everything as a massive growth opportunity. Sometimes I still think, "How the hell did I end up like this? I'm smart, I'm beautiful, I speak three languages, I travelled overseas, how the hell am I here?" But I'm not ashamed to say or think that anymore. It is what it is, and I'm proud of the life we've built.'

Her forties have seen my friend walk through fire for her children and for herself. She's made big choices and even bigger sacrifices in this decade, and she's only halfway through.

'I look forward to the next decade because my boys will be older. I am counting on their independence so I can soften into mine. I have a feeling I'll be helping other women, just like my older, wiser counsellor helped me.'

'Selfish' and 'ruthless' may have been her vehicle to emancipation, but J couldn't be further from either of those things. She is a bold and fearless hero in my eyes, the best of women, and an outstanding mother. Her future is so, so bright.

Here's what Jordana wants you to know:

- When you leave, you will struggle financially. That's a given. The first three years are difficult, but you will make it work.
- Detaching from 'the dream' is the biggest hurdle. Letting go of everything that makes you feel safe is hard. But your freedom and happiness are worth it.
- Talk to people. Tell them your situation. People are kind and compassionate. You can get a lot of real help that way.
- Prioritise your finances early. Learn a different way of doing things and make small changes. It's easy to manage money when your income is greater than your expenses. When more money goes out than comes in, you have to get savvy. It can be done.

- Second-hand everything! You will learn to love it!
- Make connections and be part of your community. Building trust with safe people is critical.
- Simplify life where you can. Keep it tight and bright.
- You don't have to have a clear vision for the future just yet. Be patient. It will come.
- Buy the new bed. Just do it.

Hip, hip, divorce!

Lise

One night, I was watching videos of relationship psychotherapist Esther Perel and she raised the importance of rituals following a break-up. She told the story of a friend of hers who, after suffering a huge relationship loss, sent invitations to her closest group of friends to gather everyone in one place so she could deliver the news one time, and one time only. No repeating and reliving of the horror story.

Over the course of the evening, the women shared quotes and poetry verses they'd saved, passages that helped them through their own heartbreaks over the years. There was wine and singing as the women shared their stories and also their subsequent good news tales – how they'd gone on to find happiness, perhaps new loves or careers – that the wheel did turn, and their friend's anguish would subside. She was not alone.

I found this so beautiful and healthy, and wondered what others had done to mark the end of a relationship, so I asked the brains trust on social media:

'We had a divorce party for my sister. We played cricket with the frozen top tier of her wedding cake and burned some of their wedding photos. Then we hit the clubs!'
~ Bec

'I had a bunch of besties over to share in too much champagne and food. They put me on an online dating site and went ahead matching me with guys. One of those guys is now my new husband! Don't get me wrong, there was the ceremonial smashing of the framed wedding bouquet, and I threw our wedding album into the pool.'

~ Kathy

'Quite some years ago, a close friend was going through a divorce. Once finalised, a group of us went out on the town and relived the hens party, but this time we called it a "Dead Chooks Night".

~ Sheri

'I went to a friend's divorce party late last year. She had a bunch of close girlfriends over, we had a few drinks and nice snacks, played a few games of "never have I ever" and then threw darts at a pic of the ex, defaced some wedding photos and destroyed her wedding dress. It was very cathartic for her and a great girls' night in!'

~ Amanda

'I bought myself a "Divorcery" gift of a nice new piece of jewellery. I was still grieving my previous life. Wasn't anything to celebrate, for me. Now, I'm all good, nearly five years on.'

~ Kerrie

'I had a fancy dress party where everyone had to come as a famous divorcée. My (now) husband came dressed as Pamela Anderson – best makeup and shaved body effort ever! Having the party closed a chapter for me. I'm a big believer in ritual and celebrating the failures along with the victories. In fairness, that experience helped me grow and become the person I am now, so that's worth celebrating right?'

~ Sue

'After an ugly split, I had wanted to trash my wedding dress in the dam, but my best friend and I ended up burning it in a bonfire while we danced around. $2999 of dress up in flames and it felt so good, so good.'

~ Paula

Attitude

One of the great things about getting older is you become emboldened. You don't have to give up on adventures, on learning new things, or trying something new ... Alongside all the other pillars of your life – just chucking something new in the mix every so often really shakes you up.

— Angela Mollard

Don't sweat it

Sarah

Remember in the late nineties when everyone had a copy of *Don't Sweat the Small Stuff* by Richard Carlson on the bookshelf? It was a collection of a hundred affirmations on ways to stop the little things causing stress in your life. A guide to calm and living in the now. It was a monumental bestseller, spending more than a hundred weeks on the *New York Times* 'Best Seller List', published in 135 countries and translated into twenty-five-plus languages. Remember it? Yeah, cool.

I didn't read it.

That's because I was nineteen and knew everything. The greatest hardship in my life was making sure I didn't get a speeding ticket fanging it to uni in my red Ford Festiva at 11.37 p.m. to then find a park, navigate the obstacle course of other sprinting students on a dark campus, then run up four flights of stairs to submit a handwritten essay in the assignment box before midnight.

Now, in my forties, I have since experienced life stress on various occasions – processed the deaths of loved ones, had an early miscarriage and realised I needed fertility treatment, even temporarily lost the ability to speak properly while thirty-two weeks' pregnant with my second child. True story. Okay, I'll quickly tell you that one . . .

I'd been working four days a week across two jobs, had a FIFO husband, and was reading a book to my 2.5-year-old toddler one night only to find while I could understand the words, I couldn't utter them correctly. For example, instead of 'ballet', 'ballot' came out. 'Giselle' became 'gazelle'. The more upset and confused I became, the worse the speech was – completely gobbledygook, and terrifying.

Thankfully, Mum was staying and took me to hospital. On admission, they suspected a stroke. Twenty-four hours of scans and tests later, the all-clear was given along with a loose diagnosis of a full-blown migraine – but without the migraine (huh?) – due to hormones surging through my body. Weird, but okay. The thing is, I would've bet my entire pregnancy management fee of $2875 it was stress that caused it – plain and simple.

Another time of trauma was when I popped into a random hair salon in an outer suburb for a $27 trim and left with a pageboy haircut that would have been fine in the 1960s if I was touring with The Beatles, but it was 2003 and I was single and unsurprisingly remained single until it grew out. It became my 'quirky hair year'. It is so hard to style hair when the tufts over your ears make you look like a confused koala.

Anyway, they are but two examples of stress – one more serious, one not-so – to showcase there's a gamut of life experiences we can individually pop in a mental manilla folder with TRAUMA on the tab.

So, when stress strikes you, to help you to return to a level of raking-a-tiny-Bonsai-garden calm, please enjoy ten affirmations honed over decades, from me to you.

1   You can only control what you can control.

Deadset, this is a gamechanger. Once you understand the only person responsible for your life – health, fitness, work ethic, and emotions – is you, a new day dawns. Other adults' emotions and behaviours are as much out of your hands as the weather.

Like, when I watch *The Sound of Music* and those nuns are banging on about 'how do you solve a problem like Maria', and name-calling her the incredibly cutting terms of a 'Flibbertigibbet', 'Will-o'-the-wisp', and a 'Clown', I want to sit them down in a pew and say 'Oi! Steady on there, penguins, only Maria can solve her own problems'. And furthermore, sending her up a mountain to be a governess to seven kids and a cranky retired naval officer should not have been their first choice. Poor thing had to make dresses out of drapes and listen to Liesl screech about being sixteen-going-on-annoying and then fall in love with a Nazi who blew the whistle on the entire von Trapp crew, who subsequently had to hide in a cemetery crypt (which I actually would have been okay with as a taphophile) and flee across snow-capped mountains in Switzerland wearing ... ponchos for warmth. If this isn't a reminder to solve your own problems and take control, I don't know what is.

2 Nothing changes until something changes.

Read it. Then read it again.

3 If you always put your needs last, why shouldn't everyone else?

Mate, come on. It's totally A-okay to walk to the front of the line.

4 If you need to quit your job, then do it.

Yes, it's 100 per cent preferable to have another role lined up, but if you are desperately unhappy in the workplace and it flows over into your personal life (spoiler alert: it always does), then leave. One of my very best friends quit her job by casually telling her co-workers she was just heading to the post office, then hot-legged it outta there and simply never came back. She was forty-six. It still puts a smile on my face to imagine people back at the office scratching their heads around 4 p.m. and saying, 'Anyone seen Nina? She left to get some stamps at 10 a.m.' Little did they know, Nina had set up camp at a high-end restaurant on a solo date to celebrate being a total badass who put herself first.

5 Pause when agitated, but let rip when you need to.

If you've paused when agitated, but are still deeply incensed, then do not bottle it up. It will seethe deep in your guts and you must, repeat MUST, release it out into the wild.

6 You don't have to smile if someone asks.

Show joy if you truly feel it. Permission granted to have a bad mood, or an ordinary day, and not pretend otherwise.

7 People are not mind-readers.

As much as telepathic communication would be an added bonus, you do have to tell people what you want/need. There is no point bitching and whingeing about a situation when you haven't even vocalised what you need, which leads me to ...

8 People can only meet known expectations.

You set the standards you expect. The aforementioned Nina taught me this one, and if I was a tattoo type, I'd get this etched onto my body in permanent ink. You want that promotion? Tell your boss.

You need to go to Pilates at 7 p.m. on Wednesdays? You tell your partner it's non-negotiable. You don't want children? Tell your significant other NOW. Not drinking alcohol anymore? Make sure everyone around you knows.

You cannot sell a secret – so scream it from the rooftops. And remember, the standard you walk by is the standard you accept.

9 Don't be too capable.

Mum taught me this one, because she was *incredibly* capable, and nobody ever asked if she needed help. Ever. This was a woman who had three daughters within eight and half years in the 1980s. My dad worked in Papua New Guinea on long rosters, and she worked as a teacher. She mowed the lawn, maintained the pool, drove us everywhere, made dance costumes, was on sports rosters, plus managed her own workload. And remember – this was in the age sans internet/mobile phones/Zoom – international phone calls on sketchy lines were the only contact she had with Dad. He would return home a hard-working hero in our eyes (and he was!), but Mum would work herself ragged sorting everything so he wouldn't be swamped in catch-up chores and the family could enjoy time together.

I didn't see it at the time, but without doubt there were people around us who knew Mum could do everything, and never saw a need to offer her assistance or a break. To this I say: no way, José.

As I've found myself in a similar situation with a husband who often works away for decent stretches, there was no way I was going down the same route as Mum. The house isn't perfectly tidy when he comes home. I will pay for outside help when needed. I work full-time. I order takeaway when tired. My groceries get delivered. I refuse to bear the load of everything ... and the guilt of *not* doing everything.

10 Let stuff slide and stop feeling guilty about it

You can't do everything. Just try waving the white flag of surrender on a few things and see if the world crumbles. If it does, I'm so sorry, but it's unlikely.

Bingo!

There's nothing quite like feeling a deep sense of belonging, whether it be to a team, a club, a community, or … an age group. It's time to fly your forties flag proudly!

We're holding up a mirror to your day-to-day existence and if you check off even one of these things in the chart on the next page, we will laugh at you and with you, and welcome you with open arms to the sorority.

At the very least, this should liven up your next get-together with the girls.

PS: Sarah is six rows down, five across.
And first row down, second across.
And seven rows down, three across.

....

Sidebar: Righto, Lise – you are one down, three across + six down, four across + seven down, four across (your son's words, remember, not mine).

....

You choose a venue because 'they play our music'.	Some of your colleagues could be your children.	You own an Aldi token.	You know the names of plants.	You own a collapsible chair.
Your old nightclub haunts are now a block of units.	You own sensible shoes, and have dabbled in arch supports.	You have an umbrella in the car.	You complain about the 'lead time' to install … anything.	You have a friend who wants to run a half-marathon.
The only dance trends you know are the Nutbush, Macarena, and Spice Girls' Stop.	You own a puffer vest and a thermos.	You pretend to be disappointed with a 5.30 p.m. dinner sitting.	It takes five full scrolls to reach your birth year on surveys.	You have a 'good knee'.
Sun sets You: It's getting late.	*Driving past a Westfield* You: I remember when that was all scrub.	*Sees Joh Griggs on TV* You: Oh, she's great, isn't she?	You somehow stuff up your neck during sleep.	You walk into trendy stores and say 'Oh, I wish I kept all my old clothes'.
You take a nap before a party.	You have an active Hotmail account.	You know at least six types of cheese.	You enter a meat tray raffle.	You turn the music down to see more clearly.
You have a signature salad you take to parties.	You moisturise in aggressive upward strokes, including elbows.	You own three different night serums – and use them all.	You have tweezers in the glove box.	You have a friend who brags about fake grass.
You are genuinely terrified of Mom jeans.	You begin to focus on functional fitness.	You have a friend who puts ice in their wine.	Your neck appears to have gills.	Your decolletage has to unfurl after a sleep.

The No List

Lise and Sarah

In May 2021, we interviewed *New York Times* bestselling author and all-round Aussie girl crush, Sally Hepworth. Her episode went on to become our most downloaded yet. Why? Because Sally cut to the chase good and proper and came clean about all the things she's saying no to in her forties.

While her list may elicit gasps of contempt from some and guffaws of recognition from others, it is undeniably one woman's middle years manifesto. Sally proudly plants her flag atop her (indoor) mountain and shouts, 'This is me! This is what I like and dislike!' She is no pretender. She is brave and frank and unapologetic about the things in life she wishes to take on versus those she chooses to side-step.

> *I say no to talking on the phone, dancing – ever – attending stand-up cocktail parties, meeting people for coffee or lunch during the week, except my Great Auntie Gwen.*
>
> — Sally Hepworth

The conversation with Sally kept going well past the podcast. She talked about how women can find it tricky saying no, but saying no to some things is what makes space for the important stuff. She urged 'no novices' to write a yes list instead – a list of the things you wish you could say yes to. Wish you could read more, find time to exercise or spend more time with friends? Then ask yourself what you can throw a no at to make space for those things.

It goes without saying these No Lists are based on an individual's current position in life. Nos can be tossed around like confetti with the right support – familial and financial. We know that, and Sally knows that. But every woman has a right to have a crack at composing her No List. Even if it's a hypothetical exercise in asking yourself – in a judgement-free, anything-is-possible world – what would you say no to?

So, here it is. With her permission and blessing (she said yes!), we give you Sally's Hepworth's iconic No List.

Things I Say No To – by Sally Hepworth

- Attending my kids' school functions/fundraisers
- Entering the school grounds for any reason
- Dropping off/picking up my kids from parties
- Cooking dinner
- Volunteering for anything or going on any committee (but I do donate books)
- Signing my kids up for extracurricular sport on a weekend
- Remembering birthdays
- Attending stand-up cocktail parties – except book launches
- Meeting people for coffee or lunch during the week (except my great-auntie Gwen)
- Entertaining at my home (apart from a few close friends and then I get takeaway)
- Going to the supermarket
- Talking on the phone (unless it's an emergency)
- Dancing
- Socialising more than once a week

- Doing homework with my son
- Playing with my kids – I facilitate play, playdates, take them to parks and so on, but I don't play hide and seek or, heaven forbid, role-play with stuffed toys
- Going on holidays with other people – anxiety!
- Preferably going on holidays at all – but I make exceptions for the sake of my family
- Feeling obliged to go outside when the weather is nice. I'm an inside person. Like an inside dog.

Ain't she a beauty? Sally has laminated her list, and we won't lie – the fact the woman has a laminator at home makes us love her that little bit more. Of course, we had to have a crack.

Lise's ManifestNo

Lise says no to	So Lise can say yes to
Full cream milk	A happy colon. Two colonoscopies later and it's clear that in my forties, dairy and I aren't great pals
Home printers	Using work resources with reckless abandon
Peeling vegetables	Additional nutrients (Jamie Oliver says so) and more time not peeling vegies

LISE SAYS NO TO	SO LISE CAN SAY YES TO
Folding socks like my mother does	Maintaining my sanity. No human should ever have to endure the French method of folding socks. The technique involves wearing the sock as a glove, peeling it back half-way, removing it carefully, doing the same to sock #2, and finally sliding sock #1 into sock #2. I'm crying just typing this. I was made to fold this way until I left home. I looked at renting an apartment at the age of nine but endured this torture until I was eighteen. Socks are now rolled into a ball, and I shan't ever go back
Sunday playdates organised by the school PC parent	Happiness. They've been at school together Monday through Friday, Mary. We're good
Sleepovers with more than four kids	Getting to know a few kids properly instead of feeling like I'm hosting the suburban equivalent of the Burning Man festival

Lise says no to	So Lise can say yes to
Pub crawls or multi-destination events	Smaller, more intimate gatherings where I get to sit on my ass with a glass of Wolf Blass and not break momentum
Holidaying in the same house as others	Enjoying my holiday and having my own space
Star Wars	Anything but *Star Wars*
Sick children at my house	A gastro-free home. If you or your kid has spewed in the last seventy-two hours, watch me walk away or spray Dettol on you like a cane toad
School information evenings	Being home with the humans I'm sending to said schools. Please email me the twelve PDF documents that I can peruse never
Carrying other people's stuff to the beach	Packing a good book and protecting my lumbar spine. Repeat after me – 'I am not your Sherpa'
Nail salons	DIY manis/pedis at home, in my undies. The year I turned forty, I realised I loathe having my nails done. I care not for it. I get bored and I can't relax my face when the electronic massage chair pummels my rhomboids

LISE SAYS NO TO	SO LISE CAN SAY YES TO
Eyelash extensions	Gaining back ninety minutes of my life PLUS not having to lie supine and motionless like Ramesses II PLUS not being a dead-ringer for Snuffleupagus

That was fun. Now, over to you.

I laugh when I think of me in my twenties: 'I'm so tired, I'm so busy'. REALLY?! You have no idea! You idiot! Once you get to your forties and you have a triage list of who needs you and what your priorities are, then I have to really protect my space, my mental health, how much I'm willing to give, and I don't want to be resentful towards people.

— Rebecca Sparrow

And for women, here's a trap, that we'll say yes, yes, yes, and feel this growing sense of desperation and panic and feeling taken advantage of, so that when we finally get to saying no, it's an explosive and emotional and slightly uncontrolled no. And we don't want to be that person, so if what we can do is say no earlier, in a calm way, we tend to avoid reaching that high.

— Yumi Stynes

Sarah's No List

Well, you've all just read Lise's grid justifying her reasons, so perhaps the first thing I'll say no to is … explaining why I say no. Here's my unapologetic list. Deal with it.

- Hosting dinner parties – my actual idea of Hell
- Complicated recipes
- 'It's wine o'clock somewhere!' jokes
- Gift registries
- Committees
- Red wine and rum
- Guilt around outsourcing help when needed
- My children – and trust me, they hear 'no' often and still know they're loved
- Shorts
- Quick baths
- Reunions
- Shellac and/or acrylic nails – a truly vicious time and money suck
- Not joining the dance floor
- Any concert with a mosh-pit
- Hair extensions – tried them, hated them
- Heels over 8 centimetres – I'm in entry-level arch support territory now
- Facebook friend requests – if I don't know you well enough to have a cuppa, it's a no
- Shaving my legs – thank you, IPL
- Children's birthday parties in my actual home – the pool and backyard only
- Inviting every child in a class to a party
- Pyramid schemes
- Professional fake tans

- Carrying massive handbags
- XOs at the end of professional emails – I know, I know, I'm a stone-cold witch
- More than one exclamation point!
- Gym memberships
- Sports bras with floating cup inserts – Dear Companies, take 'em out or sew 'em down
- Exercise pants without pockets.

Nolite te bastardes carborundorum

Lise

I love men. For the most part, I think I have a decent understanding of the male species. After all, there are three who inhabit my home – one big, two smalls. I delight in raising boys. I have a special kind of stamina for their hijinks, from jumping off verandas onto trampolines, to answering endless 'would you rather' questions that never make much sense but have me guffawing most evenings.

'Mum, would you rather go down a seven-foot halfpipe on a skateboard, or cover yourself in tomato sauce?' I can barely walk down a halfpipe without triggering vertigo, mate, so sign me up for the tommy sauce shower.

'Mum, who's your favourite koala?' I mean, how many famous koalas are there? I narrowed it down to Blinky Bill, Kenny the Koala, and Buster Moon from Sing. I landed on Buster Moon because my seven-year-old declared the others were from the olden days. He's not wrong.

'Mum, would you rather be a beetle or eat a beetle?' Been there, done that, kids. Not the *being* a beetle part, but I used to scoop up rhinoceros beetles, aged three, place the hefty bug in my gob, its front pincers carefully hooked over my lower milk teeth. When my poor mother would crouch down to offer me an arrowroot, I would open my trap in slow motion, allowing the beetle to reveal itself and hiss at her.

Sidebar: She eventually took me to a paediatric psych after I'd hidden behind the kitchen door and thwacked my older sister over the head with a broom, green with envy over her first day of kindergarten. To round out the trifecta, during a nice outing to Myer to buy a party dress, Mum asked me what colour frock I'd like, to which I answered, 'Black. I want black.' What a treasure. Turns out I had a severe magnesium deficiency, which can make kids behave like possessed, scarab-scoffing goths. At least that's what Mum told me.

So, while we're on the topic of men and *would-you rathers*, here's one for you: Would you rather have a grown-up, respectful, free-flowing, platonic chat with a bloke or suffer the pathetic, flaccid exchanges of great big, sooky, man-baby bitches who haven't figured out how to talk to women?

Yumi Stynes taught us that turn of phrase when we interviewed her for our podcast, *FORTY*. 'Great big, sooky, man-baby bitch.' I love it so much.

It refers to the type of man who:

a) is a misogynist

b) is an egomaniac

c) would fit in seamlessly as a Commander in Gilead

d) is devoid of manners and intelligence, with the EQ of a Styrofoam cup.

In my forties, my patience and tolerance for great big sooky man-baby bitches has plummeted to an all-time low. The jig is up, guys. Blessed day.

Here's the thing. I've always prided myself on my ability to engage positively with people. I like asking folks about themselves, ping-ponging convo while maintaining polite eye contact. I don't require deep and meaningful dialogue every time, far from it. I believe in the power of sizzling small talk. It's necessary in certain situations.

But there are three men (they shall remain nameless) who have tested my resolve to stay 'nice' and socially polite. These are men I've known for some time. We've been in each other's orbit, socially and professionally, for more than a decade. They know my family and some of my friends. Yet every time I see them, I am gobsmacked, and silently irate, at their inability to engage meaningfully.

A few things will happen. They'll pretend they haven't seen me. Worse yet, they'll pretend they don't know me. If I, or they, are with someone else, they'll never make introductions. All of this is often accompanied with shifty eye contact and puffed-chest body language to match their shifty, puffy egos.

If they do grace me with their attention, they'll do that thing where they scan the room for better, more important people to come along. I've had more comfortable exchanges with my chemist asking for haemorrhoid cream than with these pains in my rear.

At first, I'd always bound up to them when I saw them out, oblivious to the fact that because I didn't have a dong, they were incapable of interacting with me. My cheery disposition would be met dismissively. I readjusted my approach, realising it shouldn't be left to me to come to them. Both my father and my husband would never *not* approach a woman they knew. It's good manners to do so, right? I started hanging back, seeing how long it would take them to make their way to me, because of course they will, right? We've had barbecues in the park together! Nope.

The fury began to bubble after one defining exchange, which began in a carpark and ended in an elevator, involving Sarah.

We were attending an industry event and had parked in the bowels of an inner-city building. The nose of our vehicle pulled into a vacant spot, and just as I was yanking on the park brake, I realised we were right beside old mate, who'd arrived at the exact same time. My initial reaction? An enthusiastic, 'Oh, hi! Fancy that! How the bloody hell are you?', a bounce in my step as I walked in his direction, forgetting my resolve to hang back and play it cool.

And there it was again. The big freeze. Siberia – population me. You know those salespeople who accost you in the middle of a Westfield wanting to rub aloe vera lotion from the foothills of the Canary Islands onto the back of your hand? I was met with that same level of awkward avoidance we've all had to employ, minus the obligatory, 'Oh, thank you but I'm in a mad rush to pick up the kids. Sorry!'

Sarah witnessed it all: 'Don't you know him quite well?'

Okay, so this wasn't a figment of my imagination. I hadn't gas-lit myself. Not only had he blanked me, but he'd also blanked Sarah. What kind of man is rude to two women? We walked towards the lift and of course there he was, with his plus one. Perfect. Can't wait to be trapped in a 3 x 4-foot metal box with them. Maybe the confined environment will urge him to throw me a bone. Nope.

I was the one to toss out a figurative brontosaurus femur, again. I introduced Sarah, I introduced myself to his companion, I asked after his family. Give, give, give, give.

After that night, I swore to Sarah I would never make the first move again. Fool me once, shame on you. Fool me twice, shame on me.

I spoke to my husband about these repeat offences, searching for the why in their whack behaviour. As a naturally introverted person, he offered that perhaps they felt uncomfortable in cocktail party territory. I challenged him by pointing out they seemed quite at ease slinging their wanky espresso martinis and counterfeit charisma around the right people. And introversion doesn't equate with rudeness. Dane is walking proof of that. I have seen him have quiet conversations with all kinds of people, so no, I reject that excuse entirely.

And in true Lise style, our perfectly mature dissection of the situation quickly escalated to me screeching, 'Here's my assessment of the situation, Dane. Perhaps I'll wear a scarlet cloak and white bonnet to the next social gathering. I'll walk in, eyes downcast – that should make them feel more comfortable! They can call me "Ofdane" and cut my finger off if I dare read the drinks menu aloud!'

Dane: 'I think you need to let this go, Lise. You're spending too much energy on this topic. I get it, but you need to get over it.' (Cue: revving chainsaw.)

Thirty-five-year-old Lise would have burred up. I would have shaken my fist, referencing male privilege and a bloke's birthright to ignore women at will.

Forty-one-year-old Lise took a deep breath and let her husband's words sink in. I got up and walked myself downstairs. It was an eerily quiet descent to the laundry, where I stood between the whites and the darks, reflecting on my rage.

Why were the actions of some maddening me so? Why was *everything* infuriating me? The fact is, I'm not alone. Among women in their middle years, anger and indignation is trending. At a certain age – psychologically, biogenetically, I don't know – you get to the place when a switch is flipped. You tell yourself, 'I'm done'.

My forties are seeing me uncork long-bottled-up grievances, my tolerance for morons well and truly reaching its expiry date. I will not pander to them anymore. I will call their pathetic microaggressions out, in whatever way I can. I will not laugh away, nor make excuses for, their rudeness. For the most part, our generation has been brought up to smile in the face of almost any snub. Our younger female counterparts are much bolder and far more outspoken, and it's time we play catch-up. I'm not talking about waging a war here. Remember, I love men. I do. But I love good men. Smart men. Woke men.

Today, I feel it is inexcusable for blokes to not know how to converse with women. I count myself lucky to work among a bevy of exceptional, younger men. There is no awkwardness, no imbalance of power. They are my absolute equals, and I am inspired in their presence. I champion them, they champion me. So, men like the ones I've had to dance around? Thank you, next.

The question remains. Why has it taken me so long? I don't know. Maybe it doesn't matter so much. Either way, so many of us are letting it rip in our forties. And I love that for us.

So, to all the great big sooky man-baby bitches out there: rise up or rack off.

Nolite te bastardes carborundorum. 'Don't let the bastards grind you down.'

The new BDE

Sarah and Lise

In 2018, the acronym BDE entered the zeitgeist. And, yes, the sweary buzz phrase has had its time in the pop culture spotlight for a few years now but, since hitting forty, we've decided to claim it and rename it for our people.

BDE, or 'big dick energy', is a metaphysical state of being. It's a quiet self-assuredness; an intangible swagger that lives at the intersection of sexiness and confidence. It is a supercell of effortless cool, self-awareness and emotional intelligence.

It is, unequivocally us – women in our middle years.

But it can be abrasive to womenfolk because it infers male superiority. That said, restricting BDE to doodle-owners goes against its very nature and 'vibe', so we feel it's time to expand the lexicon.

How does 'oestrogen power play', or OPP, sit with the forty-something female hive-mind?

Here's the thing – once you hit your fifth decade, you've more than likely got it. (Sure, the oestrogen itself may be decreasing at a rate of knots but work with us here.) History repeatedly bears tales of gals who've successfully rocked an OPP. Cleopatra once dissolved a pearl in wine to prove she was richer and could party harder than a lecherous Roman general. Mary Shelley wrote Frankenstein *on a bet*. Joan of Arc, a peasant with no military training, led France to victory against England.

They are BIG examples, but OPP is within all of our reaches (thankfully) – you just have to tap in.

How about that feeling you get when you parallel park in one go, on a crowded street, while traffic's banked up? Yes, OPP! Or when you refuse to carry a handbag, thereby freeing your body from the unnecessary burden of stuff? OPP! And have you ever set an out-of-office reply stating all emails will be deleted on your return? BOOM, you are on fire.

And here's another OPP tip from us: we highly recommend walking around thinking everyone is in love with you. Let us explain.

We often joke together about the single men in the office holding us up as pillars of female perfection. Stop laughing. 'If we could just create a hybrid of Lise and Sarah – just WOW!'. We're certain they think that. In fact, we've told them that's how they should think. And Chris from Sales did laugh politely at our theory, so that's a dead giveaway. Plus, if Nick lets us use the microwave in the common kitchen first, it's because he's a little bit in love with us, right Sar? And Joel who stared a tad too long while we were all waiting in the sushi line – well, he's got a little crush, Lise, it's quite clear. Oh, how we laugh about this! It makes every interaction at work quite thrilling. And the more we joke about it, the stronger our middle-years mojo gets.

We once told a junior producer he was welcome to model his future girlfriend choices on us. 'A little bit from column A, a little bit from column B, Aaron,' we suggested, as we gestured to ourselves like giant consonant tiles on *Sale of the Century*. He stared back – a deer caught in the headlights. We're not sure if his mouth was agape because he'd never witnessed such blatant delusion and arrogance, but all that was left to do was raise an index finger to his lower chin and shut his gob for him. Another hectic OPP power move, right there.

And let's be clear – this isn't flirting. We're quite possibly the worst flirts ever. Sarah will bring up her mild astigmatism and dead pet cat stories at the most inopportune of times, while Lise quite regularly confuses aggression with affection and has been known to yell, 'RACK OFF, SHUT YOUR FACE!' as a show of her love. No, no – this is all in good-humour and jest, a reminder of what we have to offer in this world. Which, at this point in our lives, is a lot.

For us, OPP is about having spark, gumption, and choosing to look at the bright side. New bumper sticker coming in hot: 'Live your life with the confidence of a forty-something-year-old woman.'

Ask any of the blokes at work and we're pretty sure they'll agree. (Mostly because they're a little bit in love with us.)

Crying

Lise

I am crying in my forties.

Anyone who knows me will understand there are two things I don't do. Vomit and cry. I think I'm nearing twenty years without throwing up, such is my phobia of it. I'd rather be sedentary on a toilet for days at a time than hurl. A white witch once told me I'd been strangled in a past life which is why, according to her, I carry a lot of fear around my throat parts. I swear I've trained my body to process illness north to south. I realise that's potentially a load of crap but, literally, that's what I'd opt for every time.

Back to the crying. Crying is uncomfortable for me. It's not that I never cry – of course I do. I cried many tears when my father-in-law passed away suddenly. But I cried those in the shower, alone, where nobody could see me. Around my husband and his family, I'd keep it together, the emotion right there, stinging my eyes, constricting, and pulling at my throat, but rarely released.

I didn't cry when Dane proposed to me, I didn't cry on my wedding day, I didn't cry at the birth of my children. I promise I'm not a monster. Those moments were among the greatest, most powerful of my life. The emotion just doesn't come out of my tear ducts.

There are two things that do bring the water forth: music and performance. I can't explain it, but those two things are my kryptonite.

Music has always made me cry. Even as a little girl, I remember my eyes would prickle when I heard classical music. I played the violin and the trumpet through primary and high school, a real one-gal band I was, and the beauty of the compositions, how the notes and chords made perfect sense, overwhelmed me from a young age. I'd sometimes think of little boy Mozart, or young Beethoven, and be bowled over by the sheer talent they would have demonstrated. That feeling would then snowball into thinking about their parents, and how awe-struck they would have been, how proud and bewildered they would have felt to witness that level of genius. I was nine years old when these thoughts would come to me. What a weirdo.

And before you start psychoanalysing me and suggesting that maybe I was yearning for a similar recognition from my own family, trust me, I got it in spades. I remember my grandparents asking me to whip out my violin whenever friends of theirs would come for tea. My uncle John and I would jam during his weird saxophone phase at uni. At my year seven concert, my dad stood up right before my trumpet solo, the crowd silent, and proudly bellowed, 'That's my daughter!' in a thick French accent.

So, no, that's not it. Nothing deep and dark going on here. Just melodies and harmonies trying to break me.

So, a school musical? A double whammy for me. The music of Freddy Mercury *and* a cohort of child stars? R.I.P. Lise. It was my eldest son's high school show – but he wasn't even in it. Nevertheless, when the sixteen-year-old lead started belting 'I Want to Break Free' as the opening number, I was a goner.

The spiral was fast and furious in the San Damiano multi-purpose hall that evening. I took my seat, C26, beside Dane and Remy, the orchestra pit just metres away, the stage and all it promised towering before us. A pre-pubescent man–child starts tuning his bassoon and the knot in my lower abdomen begins to form.

All too soon, the conductor makes an upward motion with her baton, preparing the musicians for the coming downbeat and, oh

God, my lips are doing that weird snarling thing they do. Help! Galileo Figaro takes the stage, belts out his first phrase in a G Major and, sweet Jesus, I'm going under!

But can you blame me? Today, as a forty-one-year-old mother, I look at those young kids on stage and I am filled with admiration for them. True vulnerability at an age when awkwardness and tall poppy syndrome reign supreme. Their unadulterated excitement, their passion for performance, the exhilaration they'd be feeling, the barrier between the boys' campus and the girls' campus torn down, friendships made, the behind-the-scenes crushes that would be unfolding at a rate of knots, the innocence of following your heart's desires and just going for it – it's all so beautiful.

They were just magnificent, this motley crew of teens. They left everything up on that stage. And I left everything on my cream-coloured Seed knit. My tears, silent and private, erupting from me like the water from Tiddalik the Frog's gob. I warned Dane that the day Remy gets cast in the ensemble, let alone a lead role, I'd need to be heavily sedated. I've requested *Weekend at Bernie's* level of tranquillizers, please and thank you.

So, why are the middle years bringing all the tears? Am I alone in crying more than I've ever cried before, now I'm in my forties? What is going on?

I put it to the social media hive mind, asking them if they too were bawling over *Hamilton* tunes and Gillette ads. The answer is, I am most definitely *not* alone. Here is a list of the things that make women in their forties tear up. You may need a tissue. Or, if you're like me, you're also likely to laugh aloud in solidarity:

- any school assembly
- sports fields
- a child playing the piano
- bagpipes

- the remake of *The Lion King*
- preppies running in the cross country
- a good Facebook posting
- rugby war cries
- dance numbers
- Barnesy
- Qantas ads
- parent–teacher interviews when the teacher says, 'You have a fine, fine young man'
- *The Man from Snowy River* theme song
- Scott and Charlene's wedding
- choirs
- watching *Father of the Bride*
- Mother's Day concerts
- a homeless dog missing a leg on a TikTok video
- being serenaded by an old guy at a restaurant
- the end of *Die Hard*
- disassembling bunk beds
- Easter hat parades.

Is it because midway through our lives, we are realising that beauty really is in the small stuff? Is it because we have time to allow these feelings to come through now that we're not as focused on building our lives and careers? Is it the realisation there are no do-overs? Is this what wisdom looks like?

A friend described this time as 'the wistful years'. I wonder what she meant by that. Perhaps she's referring to the dreamy melancholy I feel when I see those drama kids perform. The realisation my turn has come and gone, so quickly. There is no regret but, my God, life seems to be accelerating at breakneck speed, and I'm floored that somehow I've become a parent sitting in an auditorium, watching my son's peers do the very things I did *just yesterday*.

'The days are long, but the years are short' – a phrase often uttered by older women, and one that would infuriate me when I was raising my babies and wishing away the exhaustion and car seat tantrums. Now those words taunt me, as I watch myself move towards the pile of size 16 hand-me-down clothing that belonged to my nephew, carefully stored in our downstairs cupboard, *for later*. But now I'm holding those Quicksilver and Santa Cruz tee-shirts and I'm walking upstairs to Remy's room. But why? Surely my boy isn't ready for these yet?

He is. Those clothes I thought would sit in that cupboard for a million years are now on his back, and I can't quite understand this because it was just last week that I thanked my sister for saving them, and vacuum sealed them *for the future*.

Another friend, also in her forties, reckons our bodies will happily find any excuse to cry now we're getting older. She says that by the time we've lived four decades, we have a hefty back catalogue of 'cryable' moments. Happy tears, sad tears, nostalgic tears – the works. This explains why older women always carry those little rectangular packs of tissues with them. My grandmother will often cry just retelling an old story. She'll say she's remembering it with love.

And so, it seems my musically induced tears and I are in excellent company. I vow to embrace the waterworks and allow myself to feel wistful every once in a while. Because maybe the weeping ambushes are, in fact, a beautiful coming-of-age story reserved for those of us who remember having to rewind the VHS tape before driving it back to Blockbuster.

If you're not quite ready for public tears, may I suggest avoiding any shows containing singing children, one-legged animals, sports tournaments and bagpipes. Nobody stands a chance against bagpipes.

Not crying

Sarah

While Lise's tears have only started to flow in her middle years, the most curious of things is happening at my end – they are drying up.

It's like the baton of free-flowing tears has been passed from me to Lise, and she's running the final leg sobbing on a sports field because someone's playing 'Chariots of Fire' through the loudspeaker with bagpipes.

It truly is fascinating because I've so admired Lise's emotional fortitude and strength in tough moments, and on some occasions even wondered if her tear ducts worked.

A few years ago, we went to the cinema to watch *Three Billboards Outside Ebbing, Missouri* – an absolute emotional rollercoaster of a tragic tale starring Frances McDormand, who won an Academy Award for her role. It was one of those flicks that left me with a puddle of bosom tears and a sore throat from repressed sobs. Not unlike the first time I saw *Braveheart* and Dad had to comfort his still-howling fifteen-year-old daughter in the carpark long after the credits rolled. It was that kind of movie.

As for Lise – nothing. Dry as a bone. A wasteland. A desert. Tumbleweeds.

Being a supportive pal, I recall asking in incredibly accusatory tone what the heck was wrong with her and why couldn't she cry LIKE A NORMAL PERSON?! She retorted that I wasn't a normal person and she felt absolutely no need to cry. All in all, a beautiful bonding moment of friendship. The Yin to my Yang.

All my life, I've been a walking teardrop waiting to fall. Laughter, happiness, surprise, shock, anger, angst, tiredness, grief – you name the emotion, I'll give you a hundred tears quick as a flash.

Lise possessed a character trait I longed for: she could argue and not bawl. Admittedly, it sounds like an odd life goal, but for any fellow criers reading this, perhaps you can relate. It was never happy nor sad tears that caused bother, it was the too many times important, serious conversations – even white-hot rages – ended unfinished due to frustrated tears impeding the ability to articulate thoughts clearly.

Many years ago, Mum offered a beacon of hope and said she used to be the same as a younger woman, but the default reaction around crying improved as she got older. I can confirm, it does.

When the specific turning point came – who knows. I think I just got sick of falling in a heap during tough conversations and made a conscious effort to stop. I now refuse to shed tears at moments requiring clarity and strength; whether for me or others.

It's odd, isn't it? While Lise is discovering crying in her forties, I'm on the other side discovering not crying in my forties ... and it's clearly revelatory for both parties.

Teach me something

Lise

If I asked you to teach me something, what would I learn?

It could be weird, cerebral, practical or hilarious. Can you shuffle cards like a pro? Can you rattle off all the Kings and Queens of England? Can you carry five dinner plates out at once, like a waitress friend of mine?

Think about the skills you've acquired over the years, what you're really good at, now in your forties, and could hands-down teach another person. I'll start – I could teach you to read music. Another girlfriend of mine? She told me she could teach any woman to wee standing up.

When I asked the same question of a group of women on social media recently, what struck me is how few cited skills related to their careers:

> I can teach you how to give a pill to a cat without blood loss. And how to do calculus.
> ~ Susan

> I could teach you the ancient Japanese craft of Kumihimo (braiding) and how to complete cryptic crosswords.
> ~ Jo

I can teach you how to make a balloon topiary tree.
   ~ Belinda

I can teach you how to catch and sex a croc.
   ~ Lynda

I could teach you how to throw a cast net to get your own bait, tie a hook on your line, catch a fish or two, fillet them and cook them up for dinner all while enjoying an icy cold beer.
   ~ Janis

I can teach you how to do the 'man jobs' around the house so that you don't have to wait six months for them to get done.
   ~ Jo

I could teach you how to make a chicken out of a tea towel. I can make a miniature wine glass out of Easter egg wrappers too.
   ~ Carly

I can teach you how to scrub up for surgery and pass instruments to surgeons.
   ~ Marika

I could teach you how to get twenty-eight prep children to sneak into a classroom silently.
   ~ Deb

I can teach you how to tie a lolly snake in a knot with your tongue. I taught four classes of year twelves last year.
~ Stacey

I could teach you how to crack a whip.
~ Shari

I'm pretty good at teaching people how to body roll.
~ Kathleen

What these women chose to share are things that make them uniquely them. The colourful idiosyncrasies and quirks they're famous for; the things that make other people laugh and start a conversation at the kitchen bench. In the tapestry of life, isn't this the stuff that really matters?

I think 'what can you teach me?' is fast becoming my favourite icebreaker with people I meet. Far juicier than the perfunctory, 'What do you do?' It's also a reminder that what we do for work does not determine who we are, let alone our worth to others. It's possibly the least interesting thing about us, really.

I mean, if someone tells me they're an orthopaedic surgeon and they can make a chicken out of a napkin, I know what I'll be grilling them about.

Naked Yoga

Lise

What on God's green earth have I done?

I've just bought a ticket to a Naked Yoga workshop. Yoga. In the nude. With strangers. In the buff. Doing yoga. Naked. I don't even like yoga. Let alone strangers.

I blame social media. And being in my forties.

It was like an out-of-body experience, as I sat on the couch, tapping through Instagram. I'd fallen upon a popular influencer's rave review of an experience she'd had in Perth. A 'naked awakening' is what she called it, as she stood for a photograph with a gaggle of women wearing bath robes, joy radiating across their faces.

For the record, I'm far from the hippy-dippy type. I'm the person who coughs around incense and struggles to show emotion. But something about those videos made me leapfrog from one profile to another, until I landed on a nude yoga website – 'This is risky behaviour, Lise. Why are you tempting fate, you loose unit?' I continued gamifying my digital dalliance – 'They never have these events in Brisbane – it's always Melbourne, Perth, Sydney. You're fine.' A huge Queensland tab winks at me from the screen. I click, convinced there's unlikely to be another workshop until 2022. The date smacks me in the face – Friday, 4 June. Two days away, in my hometown, fifteen minutes from work, on a night Dane is home, Remy is away on camp, and Max's footy training has been cancelled. A run of green lights. And now, the final frontier. I tap through to

'Buy Ticket', praying for a 'Sold Out' banner to pop up and save me. One. Ticket. Left.

Strap in, baby girl. You're doing this thing. A total of $99.50 and a PDF in my inbox later, I'd sealed my fate.

To be honest, I don't even know what I've signed up for. I must have blacked out in a moment of middle-years madness. I revisit the website. It says I've signed up for a 'powerful immersion in surrender, softening and letting go; a celebration of the sensual, female form through breath, sound and movement'. It mentions things like 'radical self-acceptance, vulnerability, and personal freedom'; that I'll be 'celebrating my naked body in a safe, candle-lit space' where I'll be invited to 'shed my clothes without being objectified or judged'.

Apparently, simply turning up is a major feat for most women; that it's 'completely normal to be fearful and anxious before the class, since being seen naked is a legitimate fear for most'. Okay, thanks, Captain Obvious. The FAQ section is punctuated by one final, poignant question that hits me straight in the guts: 'If not now, when? If not me, then who?'

Forget about it and just turn up. That's what I'll do. That's my MO until D-day.

I tell Dane about it.

'Righto, then. Well, if it's something you feel drawn to, just go for it! Sounds interesting. Will you be naked when you get home?'

He's nothing if not dependable and infuriatingly opportunistic.

The day has come. It's 5.45 in the afternoon – three quarters of an hour until go-time. It dawns on me I haven't yet secured a robe, and I must have a robe; the pre-event text from the nudey-rudey-yogi says so. I call my high school bestie, Belinda Zuccarello, who's just finished work down the road, and we decide to meet up at the local Kmart. I give Bel my brief over the phone – 'I've dropped close to a hundred bucks on this gig, Bel, so I'm not coughing up more than $15 for a kimono, you hear? Meet me in the PJ section, pronto!'

I spot her fifteen minutes later, holding up two options like her life depends on it. One is a long, waffle dressing gown. It looks stiff and costs $25. Tell her she's dreaming. The second alternative proves why Bel is like a sister to me. It's softer, lighter and has three holes in it. We know what this means, having both worked retail in our teenage years. Bel tosses the waffle abomination aside and we strut up to the cashier to ask for a discount. Down to a blueberry, thanks very much – ten bucks. High-fives with Bel, my holey kimono stuffed in my cross-body bag, as we part ways so I can join the awaiting naked sisterhood.

I pull up to a beautiful, remodelled Queenslander. It's discreet – no wacky, waving inflatable man with a sign saying 'Naked Women Inside' in sight. It's right on 6.27 p.m., and I'm positively flustered. I sign a waiver without reading it. I'm shown to a changeroom where I begin peeling off every article of clothing from my body. I'm shoving my jeans and boots into my bag, boobs flapping as I bend over muttering, 'God, grant me the serenity to accept the things I cannot change ...'

I walk into the yoga room. It's warm, bathed in candlelight, the ambiance serene, and it smells good. Fourteen women are seated in a large circle, evenly spaced. It reminds me of the 1996 cult-classic film, *The Craft*. Hail to the guardians of the watchtowers of the north, south, east and west ... pretty sure I can already see a breast.

I lay out my yoga mat between the instructor and a woman who's already starkers. I sit cross-legged, not knowing quite what to do with my eyes. Should I look at the others? I quickly scan the room for anyone I know – a school mum, a colleague, an old high school acquaintance. Clear. All strangers. I am relieved to see that eighty per cent are professional females in their forties, just like me. There are two younger women, maybe mid twenties, and a new mother in her early thirties. Women with cropped hair, women with wild, curly manes, big women, petite women, small-breasted women, others with ample bosoms – a smorgasbord of shapes, sizes and shades.

The instructor strikes a pleasant-sounding gong – and it's on like Donkey Kong. Her voice is soothing as she welcomes us and explains that we are in control of when and how we remove our robes. Some women will do so early in the workshop, others will take the full three hours to de-robe. She invites us to make the moment dramatic; to cast the covers from our shoulders in a sensual way, or at the very least with intention. I cringe a little at the performative nature of her request, hoping to slink my synthetic housecoat off in a corner and walk back to my mat, bum tucked beneath my pelvis, like a dog whose anal glands need draining.

Here's the thing. I've always considered myself to be an uninhibited person. Years of quick changes backstage at runway shows and fashion shoots meant I was well acquainted with wearing nothing but a flesh-coloured g-banger in front of designers, photographers, stylists and other models. Sarah, always ready to psychoanalyse me, pointed out the dissociative nature of those behind-the-scenes work requirements. She was right – I'd developed an uncanny ability to step outside my body and just get the job done. On set I was but a flesh machine, nothing more than a vehicle for the sample-size dress that was thrown on me and pony-stomped down a catwalk. My body was working, sure, but I wasn't necessarily connected to it. Other than in the privacy of my home, where I am wholly present and one hundred per cent comfortable, I'd never had to bare all this way before.

About one hour in, after a delightful strawberry-eating ceremony, the heaters are cranked to get-your-kit-off-already-you-prudish-binch levels. The yoga flow has begun. Most of the women are already in the nud. Me? I'm still trussed up like a Sunday roast, so firm is the tie from my robe around my abdomen. I'm saluting the sun, moving into Warrior One pose, and I'm starting to shvitz. I untie my belt, my security blanket now awkwardly draped across my nips, my yoni out for all the NASA satellites to see.

Yes, *yoni*. Get comfortable with it – I had to. I'm not one to adopt pet names for my privates, but as it turns out, yoni is a Sanskrit word for 'the womb' and 'the female organs'. Not to be mistaken with Yanny from the 'Yanny or Laurel' auditory illusion of 2018.

As per instruction, my eyes are shut, just like everyone else's. I'm about to move to Warrior Two, psyching myself up to hurl my cloak at the wall, past the oil diffuser and cluster of tealight candles.

And then, at last, I'm naked – standing outstretched like a giant starfish. I immediately lament last summer's big laser blowout. If I could pray a pube back into existence right now, I would. This is why balding men opt for a comb-over. I get it now.

I take three deep breaths to calm myself. Just as I'm starting to chill out a little, the facilitator asks us to lay on our backs and raise our yonis to the sky – '*Somebody help me; make this stop!*' I try to stay centred as I take the little lady up for a ride. Whee, there she goes!

Just when I thought things couldn't get worse, the group leader announces, 'Now, we're going to let our wild women out! This is a safe place – the doors are locked, the shades are pulled down, our eyes are shut – nobody is watching you. We're going to turn up the music and I just want you to *dance*.'

There is no scarier word in the English language to me than dance. My primitive fight or flight response kicks in – I don't think my yoni and I can do this. She continues, 'I want you to dance like you're seduuuuucing yourself!', and then the beat drops – imagine Enya with a gnarly bass. I'm desperate to see what other women are doing. If all else fails, I'll just mimic their moves. Yes, I can manage that – I'm not half bad with a choreo. But of course, the directive remains 'eyes down or closed', so I'm left to my own worst nightmares.

The lady beside me is letting rip. I know because I broke the rules and peeked. She's on her haunches, whipping her long, curly locks in sensual circles, living her best seductive life, while I'm just standing there like a stick insect moving its legs up and down on a leaf. 'Challenge yourself, Lise!' This workshop is about cultivating the strength to step out of your comfort zones and overcome irrational fear and limiting beliefs! It's about embracing your sensuality and sexuality! This is it. It's time to bust out my wild woman. Here. she. goes!

I break into a step-clap combo that would make Kath and Kim proud. It's hideous, I know it, and in my head I'm berating myself. I throw a few clicks into the mix, but it doesn't help. 'You're the worst, Lise. You are such a bad dancer! An embarrassment to wild women everywhere!'

Dancing done, and it's time for the sharing circle. Everyone's eyes are open at this point and I'm getting comfortable with being nude. One at a time, we shared why we were there, what had brought us to Naked Yoga. One woman spoke quickly and nervously about how she was perfectly comfortable being naked, but the idea of being emotionally exposed and vulnerable terrified her. Another woman on the opposite side of the room said, 'I don't want to die hating my body' – a collective nod rippling through the room. There were many women just like me, not quite sure what had brought them to this place in their lives. I said something about turning forty and wanting to extend myself in this decade, and something else about feeling like a closeted introvert in an extroverted world. I cried and I'm not sure why.

The rest of the evening progressed beautifully and meaningfully – from five-minute eye-gazing rituals, standing face to face with a 'sister' (still naked, guys) – to the 'room walk'. The music swelled – a slow, rhythmic, tribal beat – the evening's soundtrack truly magnificent. The facilitator asked us to begin pacing the room, any which way – clockwise, zigzags, whatever we felt. She instructed us to look at one another's feet, eyes low. A minute or so later, we were asked to lift our gaze to the other women's shins, then a minute after that, their thighs. Size six through to size twenty-four thighs, pale thighs, smooth thighs, muscular thighs, soft thighs. We were asked to really look at the legs of the women in front of us, beside us, and behind us; to look at their strength and recognise that these legs carried these women through their lives. It was a powerful moment, like the unique and beautiful bodies that surrounded me that night.

It's not until you are in a room completely naked among your sisters that you realise just how insignificant body shapes really are. The construct of size just didn't exist in that moment. We moved our eyes up one another's bodies – yonis, tummies, breasts, faces, eyes – 'Register what you are feeling. Do you feel deeply uncomfortable right now? And why do you feel so uncomfortable?' Our honey-toned leader reminded us that once upon a time, these sharing circles, these women's circles, existed for females to gather, talk, and share together. Seeing another woman naked was perfectly normal. They'd birth together, miscarry together, and witness one another ageing. Women have been sharing themselves and their stories since the beginning, after all.

Walking that room and witnessing those fourteen other female bodies was a truly beautiful and deeply connecting moment. So, yes, hippy-dippy turns of phrases like 'celebrating the divine feminine' and 'stepping into your feminine energy' were wheeled out that night, but you know what? It felt right, honest, and long overdue.

Was it one of the crazier things I've done in my life? Absolutely. But if you choose to associate discomfort with growth, which I do, then I'd say it was also downright transformational. Three and a half hours in the nude won't solve every problem you have or untangle the complicated relationship you may have with your body. But it's a wonderful start. Here I was thinking I'd breeze my way through public nudity, but it was one of the hardest things I've ever had to do.

It forced me to connect with the idea of intimacy – with myself, nobody else – just me; to look at my body and see more than just a sample size from twenty years ago. And it's time now, in my forties, to get to know that person, and step into who I want to be in this decade, and the next to come.

Walking out the doors of that remodelled Queenslander at ten o'clock that night, I felt lighter, elated even, a little bit in love with myself, and a whole lot freer.

I've been asked by so many people if I regretted doing it, if the vulnerability hangover got the better of me. It's a no across the board. No regrets, no nothing. Would I do it again? I don't think so, but never say never. In any case, it's made for some cracking conversations and recommendations to many, many women.

So, if there's an influx of forty-something-year-old women to that inner-city yoga workshop and they ask, 'Where did you hear about us?', there may be more than a few answers along the lines of, 'Oh, the girl wearing the Kmart robe with the holes in it.'

Isn't that the wonderful pay-off of being in your forties? Yes, you might have saggy knees and your neck's not particularly defined anymore – but that's the pay-off for knowing who you are ... and being able to give less shits, really.

— Justine Cullen

Onwards and upwards

I think as you get into your forties, you don't need to be loved by everyone and you don't need to have approval anymore, and that's really freeing. There's a beautiful freedom to that. You get rid of the 'shoulds' in your forties, you just go, 'Nah, I'm not doing the should, I'm doing what's right for me. I'm going to stand in my own spotlight and honour myself.'

— Gorgi Coghlan

Warning

by Jenny Joseph

When I am an old woman I shall wear purple
With a red hat which doesn't go, and doesn't suit me.
And I shall spend my pension on brandy and summer gloves
And satin sandals, and say we've no money for butter.
I shall sit down on the pavement when I'm tired
And gobble up samples in shops and press alarm bells
And run my stick along the public railings
And make up for the sobriety of my youth.
I shall go out in my slippers in the rain
And pick the flowers in other people's gardens
And learn to spit.

You can wear terrible shirts and grow more fat
And eat three pounds of sausages at a go
Or only bread and pickle for a week
And hoard pens and pencils and beermats and things in boxes.

But now we must have clothes that keep us dry
And pay our rent and not swear in the street
And set a good example for the children.
We must have friends to dinner and read the papers.

But maybe I ought to practise a little now?
So people who know me are not too shocked and surprised
When suddenly I am old, and start to wear purple.

Acknowledgement:

Copyright © Jenny Joseph, SELECTED POEMS, Bloodaxe 1992.
Reproduced with permission of Johnson & Alcock Ltd.

Fourteen going on forty

Sarah

The following piece was published in the *Bundaberg News–Mail* in 1995, submitted by a *certain* Grade 10 student named Sarah.

Bless my old school friend, who at thirty-nine, found her high school scrapbook, where she'd carefully cut and pasted the black-and-white article between hard-copy photos of a Sizzler birthday party and random class camp shenanigans. I can't tell you how much I want to edit the punctuation, delete the unnecessary exclamation marks of teen writing, and more broadly – punch myself in the face. Enjoy.

14 GOING ON forty

A friend of my mother's turned forty a few weeks back. She look at me and said how she wished to be my age again! She remembered the parties, the cute boys, the laughter and the carefree days of freedom! Boy ... did I have to tell her about reality!

The fourteen-year-olds of the nineties are not like the fourteen-year-olds of the sixties! Let's take the parties for example. The social gatherings of the sixties were a great chance to have an innocent good time, dancing the night away until Dad picked you up at your curfew of 10 p.m.

Today's parties can be considered as downright dangerous! Nineties get-togethers often are a great chance to do drugs, scull some alcohol and have a pretty dizzy night.

With peer pressure always looming near, teenagers today are obsessed with appearing to be 'cool', to feel accepted.

Teenagers, including boys, today will spend hundreds of dollars just to achieve the 'in' look. Why must we go so far to be considered trendy? Even I, as a teenager myself, cannot find the answer. Maybe it is because I am a victim … sucked into the never-ending world of fashion and propaganda! Try wearing a homemade dress or shirt to the disco and see what happens!

But what is perhaps the saddest difference that I had to point out to my 'envious' ageing friend was that kids my age have never known the carefree freedom that she knew as a fourteen-year-old. I'd gladly swap my Reeboks, my computer, even my own room … just to be able to walk at night up to the shop without fear of being harassed, molested, or even worse!

Teenagers today know an awful lot … we've known the facts of life for years, we know about AIDS, we know about drugs and alcohol abuse, but in learning all this, our youth has been taken away. In many ways, we are fourteen going on forty, and like my ageing friend, I wish I could be young again.

What the hell, baby Sar?!

I'm dying inside – *dying*. You never even wore homemade clothes to the disco, it was a family computer in the kitchen, you never did drugs – nor did your mates, and you carried a giant collection of Bronte sisters' novels in your schoolbag. Calm down, you dramatic lil' ratbag. And, spoiler alert: you'll get to forty and *not* want to be young again. It's great here.

Letter to a niece

Lise

My beautiful niece turned fourteen this year. I remember year nine being quite the shit-show for me in 1994, so I wanted to write her a letter, in the hope my words might land.

I wasn't sure if I'd include it here – if it even fit. But writing it has made me take stock of how far we come as women, over the course of half a lifetime. Those little flames of knowing that flicker inside of us as teenagers eventually become roaring infernos by the time we reach our forties, don't they?

The advice I give my adolescent niece still holds true for me today.

(And to add a beautifully woo-woo twist to this whole thing, turns out 1441 is a mirrored 'angel number'. Not quite sure what an angel number is.)

17 August 2021
Dear Gisele,
So here we are. You are fourteen, I am forty-one. That's a whopping twenty-seven years between us. But guess what? I remember being fourteen like it was yesterday. In fact, most days, I can't quite believe I am married with two children because my teenage years still burn so brightly in my memory. I remember what it felt like, I remember what I was doing, what made me laugh, who I could be myself with and what was important to me.

I see so much of myself in you at this age. Your hunger for independence, your devotion to your friendships, how switched on you are – with the exception that you make fourteen look rather amazing, complete with defined brow and stylish wardrobe, while I was repeatedly mistaken for a boy with a bad haircut and a back brace. The gentleman at the 7-Eleven once waved me off with a 'Have a nice day, young man'. True story.

Year nine was a really tough year for me. I went from being well-liked through primary school to finding myself lost in a minefield of girls that were now curvy and 'grown up', knew lots about things I knew very little about, and were doing far more than what I would ever have been allowed to do. I felt inferior and intimidated. They were out of my league, on so many levels.

But here's the thing. As much as I wanted to speed up my time as a scoliosis-rocking teen, I'm glad I was a 'slow burner'. Be thankful for (and mindful of) not peaking too early. It may not make sense to you as you read this, but later in life when you really come into your own, you'll be glad.

Because the girls that peak in their early teens? More often than not, they hit that ceiling of fabulousness far too early, leaving little room for them to grow, soar and hit their stride when it really counts. Your twenties! Your thirties! Your forties!

That's when the 'it' girls give way to the 'it' women. Women with strength. Women with ideas. Women with creativity. Women with guts. Women with glory. And believe me, you'll be surprised who they turn out to be.

Here's more of what I know for sure and what I would love to share with you:

- *Trust your instincts.* Make friends with them now. Your body always knows, so pay close attention. That prickly heat through your arms, that funny feeling in your gut, that pause of hesitation. They are all signs. When it comes to friends, boys and being safe, your instincts reign supreme. Don't ever feel silly. If something doesn't feel right, it probably isn't.
- *Real friends last forever.* You probably already have that one girl you know you'll always have by your side. She knows you better than anyone. You can one hundred per cent be yourself around her. You can laugh without reservation. She has your back and you have hers. My best friend, Belinda, and I have been inseparable since year eight. Sarah and I have become like sisters in the space of six years.

  We've had our ups and downs, disagreements, the usual. But years on, they are both still here, and our friendships are stronger than ever. Treasure these connections. Know who those people are. There won't be many like them.
- *Let your heart guide you.* It whispers, so listen closely. This applies to relationships, life, and career goals. Know yourself. Know what you bring to any given situation. Know your strengths, your talents, what makes you unique and what makes you incredible. Back yourself. We're always told to make smart decisions and think with our heads. But listening to our hearts is equally important. That's where your truth lies. That's where your happiness lives.

  When I was living in New York, I was in a relationship with a man that ticked so many boxes. But something wasn't right. He didn't make me as happy as I knew I wanted to be. My head said yes – on paper he was perfection – but my heart said no. I knew my life wouldn't look the way I'd always imagined it if I chose him. I ended up leaving my work, leaving my apartment, leaving the country, leaving everything. It was a huge leap of faith. But I listened to my heart and my heart didn't let me down. Dane showed up not too long after that.

- In terms of work and career? By God, listening to my heart has been paramount for me. When people said no, I kept pushing. When people told me the job I wanted simply didn't exist, I didn't listen. I've analysed my strengths, looked closely at what makes my heart sing, mixed it all together and voila! Yes, it's taken time, but my heart has guided me to where I am now. If you have a goal, go for it. Risk something or forever sit with your dreams. Ask questions. Make smart plans and just do it!

- *Be kind.* Make this your default switch. Because kindness is everything. Be kind to the kid that's a bit different. Be kind to the checkout assistant at Woolies. Ask people about themselves. Show interest in their lives, no matter who they are. Kindness breaks down barriers and creates opportunity – believe me. Carry this with you. It will serve you well.

- *Don't let others intimidate you.* I really shouldn't swear in this sort of letter, but I'm going to. Everyone's shit stinks, Gisele. So don't ever let someone intimidate you. Yes, you will come across people with better jobs, better houses, better cars, better prospects … but if they are getting off on intimidating you it's only because they recognise the greatness in you, and they're scared of it. That's the truth.

- *Talk*. One of the things I value the most as a female is my relationships and conversations with other women. Women are knowledgeable. Women know. Women understand. Good women won't judge but they will listen, and they will advise without preaching. Find those women, Gisele.
- Real women won't be afraid of telling you the good, the bad and the ugly. 'Friends' who only paint a picture of perfection? Forget them. Find your tribe of brave females that will admit and share when things are tough, when things feel scary, when failure has occurred. Find the girls that will celebrate your successes without a hint of jealousy. Be the girl that is honest and open about her feelings. Because lying and pretending is exhausting and just not worth it.

Gisele, you are such an engaging, intelligent, alluring, interesting, captivating person. The future holds exciting things for you, and I can't wait to watch in the wings. I know you probably can't wait to be done with school. I remember that feeling so well. But isn't it a wonderful thought that some of the best days of our lives haven't yet happened? Imagine what you are yet to experience, what you are yet to achieve!

You are a stunning young woman, Gisele. You are striking, so people are naturally drawn to you. Just remember to trust those instincts and be selective with who you let into your inner circle. I've worked with 'beautiful people' for most of my career and let me tell you something – people are prettiest when they talk about something they really love with passion in their eyes. You are more than what you look like. You have brains, humour, and kindness to match. Don't ever forget that. You are the whole package. Go get 'em!

Xo Lise

What do you wish you'd known before turning forty?

Lise and Sarah

I was braver to say no to things that weren't right. And I was braver to jump into things that I wanted to do without waiting. I think if I went back to my twenties, I would just be much ballsier. If I could go back and change anything, that's what it would be.

— Sally Obermeder

You're not the beginning and the end of the world. It does go on without you and without your input, and you can either find that out by taking baby steps backwards from some of your responsibilities, or you can find that out when you are hauled out of your life kicking and screaming and it just has to go on without you. One way or another you're going to find it out ... Just understand that there are very few things that only you can do ... I wish I had had that module installed in my brain a lot earlier ... I don't have to be the project manager for everything ... If you aren't making it happen, it doesn't happen and if you want it done right you got to do it yourself – those are attitudes that will keep you in chains.

— Julie Goodwin

I want to go back to my thirty-year-old self and just say play bigger, start earlier, and don't give a shit. Because that's certainly how I feel now.

— Mel Browne

Everything you do up until your forties, you are going to be able to utilise. That small stint you spent working in a café, the summer you spent working at a charcoal chicken shop, that time you played water polo or studied beauty therapy, and even that crazy thing you did in your twenties, it will all come full circle. You'll be surprised at how much you grab a hold of when you enter your forties.

— Emmylou MacCarthy

I'm forty-three now and I've got to say, these are the best years of my life. Don't get me wrong, I've had some hard moments in the last couple, in particular, but … anyone listening who's heading towards their forties or in their forties, there's just this sense of peace and calm about who you are and I think you're able to connect to people and the things you want to do in your life. You're very good at saying no, you're so much better with boundaries, but I'm discovering I'm saying even more yeses to adventures and therefore, as a result, my life is super dynamic and lots of fun.

— Taryn Brumfitt

When I turned forty, it was like, I wanted to follow my heart. People say, 'Follow your heart!' And my heart led me to hell. So, now I don't follow my emotions. My emotions need to be in the back seat with a seatbelt on and controlled. I use my mind, my logic, counsel, and my emotion comes secondary. Instead of

When you turn forty, there does seem to be a switch that's flicked and you become aware of your mortality. I suddenly felt like, 'Oh yeah, that's right, life does not go forever and I'm probably roughly halfway or, like, middle aged, right?' And then I realised, 'Oh yeah, wow, that forty years went so fast, and I guess the next forty will go fast, and so I need to be really clear about what I want to do with the next forty. What do I want to do with this life because it doesn't last forever?'

— *Meshel Laurie*

saying, 'I feel like doing this!' – 'feeling like' is not always that wise ... I often say to people ... 'Play the tape. Play the tape'. Is that the end result that you want?

— Andre'a Simmons

Probably a great lesson that my grandmother taught me ... boy, it has held me in good stead to this day, and that is, 'not everyone is going to like you, darling'. You just have to be at one with that.

— Catriona Rowntree

I would tell my forty-year-old self, don't put things off and don't be afraid of trying new things.

— Paula Joye

What do I wish I knew before turning forty? I wish I'd known earlier that the idea of getting older is not only about decline. That's BS. The strength and the power women have as we get older when we're not so focused on being liked, or the male gaze, and we can actually focus on 'What am I here to do?' We can *create a lot of space and lot of impact. This time can be a time for us to really knuckle down into who we are – imperfections and all.*

— Kemi Nekvapil

You don't have to have it all by the time you're forty. I love the saying 'everything will be okay in the end, and if it's not okay – it's not the end', and I truly believe that. I've learned to pause when agitated and be a lot calmer. In my thirties, I was probably a bit more panicked, more stressed, a harder person to deal with, but now? That's okay. Everything will be okay.

— Samantha X

We posed this same question to other women in their forties through social media, and they delivered in spades:

- The best years are coming.
- What a liberating, self-assured time it is. A wonderful key change.
- Your kids can only sit on your lap for a cuddle for a very short period of your life. Make the most of it.
- Unexpected hair, and yes, those legs are gorgeous – show them off!
- That I'd known my self-worth so I could start loving myself earlier.
- That I'd become the parent in the parent/child relationship, looking after and advocating for my mum.
- Career changes after forty are possible. Go for it.
- That a lot of people are not as smart or with it as they appear to be.
- Speak up – your questions are valid.

- You can keep changing! You're not 'all grown up', it's not all over.
- Neck cream is totally a thing.
- Now's the time to quit bad habits before they hit you on the head.
- Losing five kilos will dramatically help with hip, ankle or knee pain.
- Carbs will be your greatest enemy.
- You're stronger and braver than you realise.
- Never stop learning.
- When someone shows you their true colours, believe them.
- Don't wait. Do it now.
- Don't worry about what others think. They're too busy focusing on their own lives to care.
- Don't get bogged down in things you can't control.
- Don't waste time on cheap champagne.
- Mammograms are free for women over forty, not fifty, as advertised.
- Wear sunscreen every day.
- That ending my marriage was the best decision I ever made.

The bucket list

Lise

It was a Saturday night; Dane had the pizza oven fired up, one of the boy's little mates was over for a sleepover, and one of my besties dropped in for impromptu arvo sav blancs – life was good.

At some point, we grown-ups started chatting about our respective bucket lists for the second half of our lives. It made me stop and *really* consider what I want the next decades to include so, although my list is still quite rudimentary, here we go:

- Great Ocean Road on the Harley Davidson with Dane
- Tasmania – hikes plus cheese plus wine
- Some sort of retreat with my mum and my sister
- Manhattan with my two boys once they're both 21.

Then I got curious. What did other women I know want to be, do, or see in the remainder of their lifetime? Their social media replies came through thick and fast:

- Successfully host a dinner party
- See a Renoir painting up close
- Go on a hot air balloon ride
- Grow roses in my garden
- Walk the Kokoda Track in PNG for my granddad
- Take six weeks off work and walk the Camino with a girlfriend

- Compete in a triathlon
- Backpack around Canada
- Head to Glastonbury with the kids
- Start my law degree
- Learn ballroom dancing
- Sky dive
- Experience a White Christmas in NYC
- Live in the south of France for three months
- Travel from Esperance to the Kimberley with no timeframe
- Swim with whale sharks
- Stay in an over-water bungalow
- Visit Dick and Angel at Chateau de la Motte-Husson from *Escape to the Chateau*
- Watch the sunrise over Uluru
- Take my mum to Europe
- Sail around the Whitsundays
- Go to the Country Music Awards in Nashville
- Take High Tea at Claridge's
- Drink prosecco on the Greek islands
- Have a solo-hiking holiday
- Climb Kilimanjaro
- Go to the Australian Open
- Watch the Formula 1 in Monaco from a house above the track or from a super yacht
- Attend the Oscars
- Build my dream home
- Visit Giraffe Manor in Kenya
- A bucket (Okay, wise guy, thank you!).

The term 'bucket list' came from screenwriter Justin Zackham, who developed a list of things he wanted to do before he died. Years later, his bucket list became the title of the 2007 film starring Jack Nicholson and Morgan Freeman, telling the story of two old men with terminal cancer who want to live it up before they die.

So, is the idea of a bucket list morbid? It's an exercise that asks us to contemplate our own death, so yes, maybe it is. The rebel in me sometimes thinks the notion of a bucket list is moronic and should be wiped from our collective vocabulary. That escalated quickly but hear me out. What if a bucket list is just a socially acceptable way to express our heart's desires because they're framed in the face of our death? (Wow, Lise, you're a ray of sunshine today.)

Here's an example:

Scenario 1

Jane: I really want to learn hip hop dancing.

Gillian: Why on earth would you want to do that for? You're a lawyer who wears sensible shoes, for God's sakes, Jane!

Scenario 2

Jane: Learning how to dance hip hop has always been on my bucket list.

Gillian: You're an inspiration to all of us, Janey, and a hoot to boot! (Starts playing 'Get Ur Freak On' by Missy Elliott.)

Firstly, I feel Gillian needs to be weeded from Jane's friendship garden. What a two-faced cow. Secondly, why shouldn't Jane's own

The forties are so, so great because I think the twenties are just full of angst … and then your thirties are very driven by ego, and I think women and men, ego sits in front of your thirties, and then you hit forty and that ego starts to fade. And that's really relaxing. And you're just really in a great, great wheelhouse as a forty-year-old woman. I think the forties are a fabulous decade.

— Paula Joye

pleasure and curiosity be reasons enough for her to take action? Why does she need to wheel out her own expiry date as justification?

Anything that lights a fire in your belly, go give it a go. Don't ever let someone talk you out of trying something if you really want to give it a go. It's not your age, it's not your weight, it's not what you look like, it's not where you live … this is your gift, right here.
— Emmylou MacCarthy

Also, I am Jane. I've always, always wanted to be a back-up dancer, even though dancing terrifies me. Please don't laugh. Actually, I don't care if you do. Sure, I've never had dance training in my life, so being in a pro squad is unlikely to happen in this lifetime, but will I sign up to a class and learn a choreography complete with rib isolations and step-ball-changes? Yes, I will. Because I must. And I'll be damned if I find myself on my death bed wishing I'd been honest and brave enough to chase the things that light my soul on fire.

I saw a social media post not too long ago that suggested a way of reducing the bucket list concept into bite-sized chunks. Twelve in twelve. One actionable must-do item per month for a year. I like it.

First up – figure out what the hell a step-ball-change is.

Whatever it is that works for you, I say chase your joy with reckless abandon beyond the tick of a list. Life is too short. We know that now we're at the midway point of our lives, right? If you want to try something, just own that you want to try it. And to hell with the Gillians of the world who may think you've lost the plot. They can shove their sensible shoes where the sun don't shine.

Maga manifesto

Lise

Rebecca is an old colleague and dear friend. Anyone who has the good fortune of meeting Beck will comment on one of three things – her radiant smile and contagious laugh, her immediate warmth, and her exquisitely eclectic fashion sense – she worked with a myriad of famous Aussie songstresses as a stylist, and has been known to wear vintage ball gowns from her archives to Coles. Beck is possibly the most unique woman I've ever met, her approach to life equally extraordinary.

Beck is forty-five years old and a mother to three daughters. Her eldest recently graduated from biomedical science and has been offered a suite of medical scholarships. The apple doesn't fall far from the tree – Beck had studied biochemistry and microbiology, with more book smarts than most. This information is pertinent because what happens next in her story doesn't necessarily follow the script.

When Beck was thirty-four years old, her father passed away from an aggressive cancer. Despite being numb with grief, she couldn't ignore the persistent and undeniable brushes she was having with the spirit world. It was an ability she'd had from an early age; one she'd turned away from for decades. The tussle continued for a few more years, and then, on the cusp of turning forty, she decided to run towards it.

Beck is now a sought-after intuitive reader and energy worker. She's not in the business of future predictions, or trickery. Sarah and

I will often tap into Beck's wisdom and have affectionately called her our 'white witch'. Meeting up with her feels like a universal, energetic reset. You get right with yourself when you chat with Beck. She has this beautiful way of offering up new ways of seeing the world, and your place in it.

She nudged us to set a meaningful business intention; she encouraged us to use our voices, confirming we were on 'the right path'; and she taught us not to be afraid of life's seasons.

In our forties, we've turned to Beck again, wanting more White Witch Wisdom around this very topic. Beck explained that a woman's life is in four parts – Maiden, Mother, Maga, Crone. Each life season has a corresponding rite of passage – birth, childbirth/career birth, menopause, retirement. She went on to say that in our fifth decade, we were entering our Maga phase – the autumn season of a woman's life – the harvest. She spoke excitedly about 'arriving at Self' in our middle years, and how the Maga archetype was a force to be reckoned with.

We liked the sound of this Maga woman a great deal. We asked for more Maga magic, to expand our own frameworks and attitudes around ageing. And perhaps yours.

Beck delivered in spades.

Hello darlings,

The Dalai Lama has a famous quote that reads, 'The world will be saved by the western woman'. I would add to this that the world will be saved by the middle-aged western woman.

So, here she is in all her glory – Maga. I'm in love with her and am allowing her to move into these bones of mine more and more.

— Beck

Who is Maga?

- Maga, or the perimenopausal woman, is the beginning of *becoming power*. She has come full cycle, through the maiden and matriarch archetypes.
- There is a Native American saying that shares: 'At menarche, a young woman *enters* her power; through her menstruating years she *practises* her power, and at menopause she *becomes* her power.'
- She has moved fully into her skin, present and embodied, and is ready to take up the space she needs. The suppression of feminine power has made her invisible for generations, but her role now in this world is to be seen as a powerful space holder.
- She is less interested in things to *do* as she is in things to *be*.
- She ages *gratefully*, through her spirituality and connection to her own heart. Not fooled by society's obsession with youth, she has no need to look back, and knows all things happen now, in the present. As her body travels through the natural ageing process, she knows that her spirit and essence will animate and grow stronger.
- She has dropped out of her *knowledge mind* and into her *knowing heart*. She trusts her intuition.
- She is moving away from *hard work* towards *heart work*.
- She has released the need for external validation and exclusivity. Her lived experience has shown her that nothing outside of her (partner, children, house, car, and so on) could truly define her. Finally, to her own self she is true, and thus deeply inclusive.
- Through her integrity and by facing her own true north, she

chooses to serve with her gifts and talents. She leads from wisdom.

May you allow the power of Maga to awaken in you.

Forty things we wish we knew before turning forty

Sarah and Lise

1 Strength and weight training are a must.
2 Will what worries you now matter in five years? If yes, carry on. If not, give it five minutes then move on.
3 If a dress code is unclear, just wear black.
4 Do not sit with resentment. Express what's bothering you early.
5 Never trust a bloke with a shark-tooth necklace.
6 Being busy is not a marker of success: it can be a red flag. Calm, slow moments are vital.
7 Sleep when you're tired; stretch when you're tight; stop eating when you're full.
8 A jar of pesto and a packet of pasta in your pantry will save you every time.
9 You have permission to recalibrate and dream new dreams.
10 When in doubt, say, 'Let me think about that' – it'll buy you time while letting the other person know you're taking the request seriously.
11 Don't waste a single second loathing your body.
12 No one needs a one-hour meeting.
13 You need new bras every year.
14 When someone dies, always speak their name to those they loved.

15 There is no greater joy than being home, showered and in pyjamas by dusk.

16 Reassess the booze.

17 Your life partner will change, and so will you. You are not meant to stay the people you were in your twenties or thirties.

18 No more doctor-hopping – find a good GP who listens to you.

19 Pay attention to the people who don't clap when you win.

20 Streamline and simplify your life. Purge your stuff. Establish order.

21 Forget keeping up with the Joneses – comparison is the thief of joy.

22 Automate your savings. Set up a basic round-up app.

23 Look after your skin long before you think you'll need to.

24 Don't write off old people – they were your age once.

25 Your pleasure shouldn't take a backseat.

26 Never make a decision when angry, a promise when happy, or grocery shop when hungry.

27 Fiddle leaf figs are temperamental bastards.

28 There's no such thing as 'dressing for your age'.

29 Share the mental load if you can. Install school and sport apps on both parents' phones.

30 Never buy leggings with seams along the crotch.

31 Don't ask a grieving person what they need, just take action.

32 Always listen to your gut and live by the three-second rule: ask yourself a question and reach a yes or no answer in no more than three seconds.

33 Buy good-quality pots, pans and knives.

34 Asserting yourself does not make you a difficult woman.

35 Ugg boots are worth the investment.

36 Take note of how many times you needlessly apologise in a day.

37 Travel whenever you can.

38 Never feel guilty for trapdoor-ing or smoke-bombing from large gatherings.

39 Always have tweezers in your glove box.

40 Start writing this book early. Nope, earlier than that. Earlier again. Bit more.

FORTY, the podcast

Alison Brahe-Daddo, former Australian Supermodel, 8 October 2020

Sarah Wilson, Author and Climate Advisor, 15 October 2020

Ada Nicodemou, Actress, 22 October 2020

Yumi Stynes, Author and Media Personality, 5 November 2020

Emmylou MacCarthy, Televison Presenter and Author, 16 November 2020

Gorgi Coghlan, Television Presenter, 26 November 2020

Shelly Horton, Journalist and Television Presenter, 3 December 2020

Paula Joye, Magazine Editor and Digital Creator, 10 December 2020

Kathy Lette, Author, 1 February 2021

Lisa Cox, Writer and Media Diversity Professional, 8 February 2021

Angela Mollard, Journalist and Columnist, 22 February 2021

Narelda Jacobs, Journalist and Presenter, 1 March 2021

Taryn Brumfitt, Film Director and Author, 15 March 2021

Julie Goodwin, Chef and Media Personality, 22 March 2021

Mia Freedman, Co-founder of Mamamia, 19 April 2021

Mel Browne, Finance Expert and Wellness Advocate, 21 April 2021

Kemi Nekvapil, Coach, Speaker and Author, 26 April 2021

Rebecca Sparrow, Author, 17 May 2021

Andre'a Simmons, Founder of Australian Anti-Ice Campaign, 24 May 2021

Sally Hepworth, Author, 31 May 2021

Sally Obermeder, Company Co-founder and Media Personality, 7 June 2021

Catriona Rowntree, Television Presenter, 14 June 2021

Samantha X, Author and Escort, 21 June 2021

Shanna Whan, Founder of Sober in the Country, 12 July 2021

Megan Daley, Teacher–Librarian, 19 July 2021

Meshel Laurie, Comedian and Author, 26 July 2021

Dr Naomi Potter, British Menopause Society Specialist, 2 August 2021

Frances Whiting, Columnist and Author, 9 August 2021

Beth Macdonald, Business Owner and Blogger, 18 October 2021

Urzila Carlson, Comedian, 25 October 2021

Emily Jade O'Keeffe, Radio Presenter, 15 November 2021

Acknowledgements

General thanks

First and foremost, our utmost thanks to the women within these pages who trusted us to tell their stories and include their words to share with the world. You made this project much bigger than the two of us, and we're so grateful. We'd rattle off your names, but many of you are under pseudonyms like some kind of 40+ year old spies, so we shan't blow your cover.

Next, our manager and friend, Claire Savage, who knew there was a book in us long before we did. If it weren't for Claire's gentle prodding to meet looming deadlines, we'd still be procrastinating our way through endless *Kath & Kim* memes and re-watching *Schitt's Creek* 'for inspiration'.

To the Echo Publishing team, who swooped into our lives and offered us a book deal mere weeks after the *FORTY* podcast launched: thank you. What a life-affirming experience this whole project has been. Tegan, Emily, Diana, Juliet and Lizzie – as debut authors who had no idea what the heck we were doing, you held our hands and stepped us through this initially terrifying and insurmountable task with nothing but positivity and encouragement.

And to our editor, Joanne, whose expertise picked up glitches and guided us to cherry-on-top territory. Even though the margins came back relatively unscathed, you've probably read this book more than us. What an effort.

To the Those Two Girls audiences we've chatted to and with over many years on radio, podcasts, events, social media and emails, we appreciate you more than you'll ever know. It's because of lending us your time and ears and support that we've been able to change our career trajectory and have some pretty dreamy jobs, including now being published authors.

Oh, did you think we were finished? But wait, there's more …

Acknowledgements – from Lise

To Sarah – we bloody did it. Here's to sharing our fifth decade and beyond together, ageing gratefully side by side.

To Uncle John – the very best advisor, mentor, business Yoda and friend we could ask for. Your wisdom and insights are invaluable to us. We couldn't do any of this without you.

To my sister, Fred – you were the first to read my pieces. Having you laugh, cry, unpack and react to my writing is everything to me. Your opinion matters the most.

To Belinda Zuccarello – whose veranda I sat on and whose phone I blew up too many times to count when feelings of doubt crept in. You will always be my true north.

To my parents – parts of this book cracked me wide open. Thank you for catching me, talking things through, and answering my thousands of questions. From the very first story I scribbled down in my 1986 Year One classroom, you've never stopped believing in my abilities. Your faith in me is my superpower. *Merci. Je vous aime.*

Remy and Max – my noisy, busy, gel-gun-wielding, stilt-walking, footy-throwing, ladder-jumping, dirt-bike-riding muses. Your love, humour and boundless energy are my fuel. You are the making of the 41-year-old woman I am today. I hope I can make you proud.

And finally, to Dane. You bellowing, 'LEAVE YOUR MOTHER ALONE!' has been the soundtrack of this book. Your belief in everything I do is the greatest, greatest gift of my life. My fierce and steadfast champion. I love you like fireworks.

Acknowledgements – from Sarah

To be honest, I've completely run out of word-puff so will keep this short and sweet. The intensity of my emotions is equal to Lise's spiel above, but I left descriptive writing on page 299.

Est. 1980

Mum, Dad, Rach and Jen: I didn't get a choice to be related to you all, but I absolutely won the Lotto. Like, the once-a-year $80 million draw level that everyone buys a QuickPick in but only one lucky sod ends up taking home the entire haul. Well, I'm the lucky sod.

Est. 2008

Wills: We *did* get a choice to be related, and I pat myself on the back quite regularly for deciding to marry you. And not just because you're a mango farmer and I get free mangoes for life, but that is part of it. You also have great hair.

Est. 2011, 2013

My daughters: Hands-down the happiest days of my life were when you were born. You continue to bring me joy but no, you're not getting a phone. I consider this book a legacy of sorts and love the thought of you as adults able to read words from your grandmother and aunts and my best friends about this period in our lives. May it bring you comfort and pride in years to come.

Sarah Wills and Lise Carlaw

Est. 2014

Lise: What an absolute boon you've been to my life. You've changed everything for the better. Let's have at least a decade rest until our next book.

In the spirit of reconciliation, we acknowledge the Traditional Custodians of Country throughout Australia and their connections to land, sea and community. We pay our respects to Elders past and present and acknowledge the rich and ongoing culture of storytelling of Aboriginal and Torres Strait Islander peoples.